Keto Diet For Beginners 2021:

Achieve Rapid Weight Loss and Burn Fat Forever in Just 21 Days with the Ketogenic Diet - Lose Up to 21 Pounds in 3 Weeks

Tyler MacDonald

Table of Contents

Introduction

Using this book as a guide will help you to easily make a lifestyle change that millions of others have already made. You will be amazed at how great you look and feel by eating foods that are delicious, healthy, and natural. You will discover its physical and mental benefits, and you will unlock a constant supply of energy.

In order to be successful with the keto diet, you will have to understand the basics of your body and how dieting works.

Many people have tried South Beach, Mediterranean, low-fat, low-calorie, Paleo, Weight Watchers, and so on. Most of them will require you to starve yourself, eat boring foods, strictly keep track of numbers, or go through a bunch of phases. The problem with the vast majority of diets is that they aren't always nutritionally sound, and they are definitely not all that satisfying. This makes them unsustainable and possibly unsafe. They aren't conducive to a happy lifestyle.

The most successful diets tend to be those that reduce your consumption of carb-rich foods. Studies have found that those who reduce their carb intake and don't change their calorie intake will lose more weight than those who follow a low-fat diet and reduce their calories. Low-carb dieters will often see improvement in their insulin, blood sugar, and triglyceride levels.

The reason for this is the way in which your body works. When carbs are consumed, your body turns them into glucose, which raises your blood sugar. Your body then produces insulin to reduce your blood sugar levels. Years of this will cause your body to have to produce more insulin. This can cause you to become insulin resistant, which can turn into type 2 diabetes.

The ADA has found that one in three adults in the US are prediabetic, and one in ten have type 2 diabetes. CDC says that the number of obese adults in the US has spiked since the 1980s from 15% to 35% of people aged 20 to 74. This is largely due to a change in diet.

The USDA made their first dietary guideline release in 1980, and they said that fats and oils needed to be heavily reduced as well as sweets. They said that carbohydrates should make up most of your daily food consumption. They soon released the Food Pyramid Guide, which put carbs at the bottom and recommended that you eat six to 11 servings a day. They also told us to eat two to four servings of fruit. Decades later, this guideline is still the framework for the US consumer education messages from various government organizations.

Healthy carbs are still suggested for diabetics instead of reducing carbs. If carbs are made up of mostly sugar, and sugar is what caused the disease, why should carbs be the main part of your diet? There are no essential carbohydrates. The body is able to create its own glucose through gluconeogenesis.

On the flip side, you have no doubt heard that monounsaturated and saturated fats cause heart disease, among other health problems. In just the last decade, dozens of studies have found similar conclusions: these types of fats have no effect on heart disease risk.

The majority of fats are essential for our health; this is why we have essential fatty acids and essential amino acids. Fats are a more efficient form of energy and contain around nine calories. When the majority of your diet is made up of fats, your body will adapt and use stored fats for energy, but more on that later.

This book is here to provide you with the information that you need to succeed with a ketogenic diet through simple cooking to achieve long-term success and weight loss.

Chapter 1: Low-Carb and High-Fat

The easiest way to explain the ketogenic diet is that it is a diet that is high in fats, low in carbohydrates, and a medium consumption of protein. This diet became a popular way to treat refractory epilepsy in children. This diet causes the body to burn fat rather than carbohydrates for its energy source.

The carbs that many people eat get converted into glucose. The body then transports it around, and it is important to fuel the brain. If our bodies don't have a lot of carbs, the liver will convert fats that have been stored in the body into ketone bodies and fatty acids. These ketones will go to the brain and replace the glucose. These raised ketones are what helps reduce the frequency of seizures related to epilepsy.

About half of the children who were put on this diet had a reduction in the number of seizures they had. The good news is the effects continue after they returned to their normal diet.

The classic keto diet will contain about a four to one ratio by weight of combined carbs and protein to fat. This can be done by getting rid of foods that are high in carbs, such as pasta, sugar, bread, grains, fruits, and vegetables that are starchy. This diet also increases the consumption of cream, butter, and nuts that are high in fat.

Most of the fats that are found in foods are LCTs or long-chain triglycerides. What's crazy is that MCTs or medium-chain triglycerides are the ones who are more ketogenic. Many people who follow the ketogenic diet use coconut oil a lot because it is high in MCTs. They might also choose to buy MCT oil and put it in their coffee for an added boost each morning.

Every person's needs and body will be a bit different; what macros makeup in a normal keto diet is normally 60 to 75 percent of their calories will come from fat, 15 to 30 percent comes from protein, and five to ten percent are from carbs.

After you've been on the diet for a few days, your body enters what is called ketosis, but we will go into that later. This is when the body begins using the fat that has been stored and eating it for energy.

Even though this diet was created to treat epilepsy, people began noticing it was useful in losing weight. Basically, when you eat carbs, your body will retain fluid so it can store the carbs for energy. When you aren't consuming as many carbs, you will lose all the water that has been stored.

Most people who begin this diet want to lose weight. This diet is great for that because it gets rid of all the stored fat in the body.

This diet seems hard to stick with because it does restrict many foods, but there are many creative ways to ensure you don't miss out on tasty meals. If you can stick with it, you are going to notice your waistline beginning to shrink.

There are many foods out there that target keto dieters. FATBAR is the first one to come to mind. Their snack bars contain 200 calories, 16 grams of fat, and four net grams of carbs.

If you love coffee and love having a vanilla latte each morning, you can start drinking bulletproof coffee instead. This is normal coffee with some MCT oil and butter mixed in.

Being able to maintain a low-carb, high-fat diet is essential for weight loss. It helps reduce risk factors for Alzheimer's, stroke, heart diseases, diabetes, and more. This diet encourages you to eat whole foods such as healthy oils and fats, veggies, fish, and meat. It reduces all the processed foods. This diet is one you can keep doing long term and be able to enjoy it. Why can't you enjoy a diet that lets you eat eggs and bacon?

Carbs get turned into sugar when digested, and this causes, crashes which will lead to cravings for carbs. This cycle will cause insulin spikes and could lead to prediabetes and type 2 diabetes.

Studies show that this diet can help people lose weight, improve their energy levels, and stay satiated for longer. This increased satiety and energy come from the calories you are getting from fats. These fats get digested slowly and are dense in calories. Dieters who follow this diet will consume fewer calories since they feel fuller longer and don't get hungry as often.

Beginning a Keto Diet

Many people will shorten the ketogenic diet to just keto. The word keto is derived from the fact that your body will create fuel molecules called ketones. These get used as an alternative fuel source for the body when glucose is in short supply.

When you eat a few carbs, these ketones get produced. This holds true when you keep your protein intake to a moderate level. Too much protein can be turned into sugar.

The liver will create these ketones from the stored fat in your body. Our bodies will then use these ketones as fuel in different parts of the body along with the brain. The brain uses a lot of energy each day, but it can't fun off fat. It can only get energy through ketones or glucose.

When following a keto diet, your whole body will change its fuel supply to run almost completely on fat. Your insulin level will drop, and fat burning will increase. It will be easier for the body to access the fat stores in order to burn them. This is great when you want to lose weight. There are other benefits that aren't as obvious such as mental alertness, less hunger, and more energy.

How Low is Low-Carb?

This diet works best when you consume very little carbs. The less you eat, the more effective it is going to be for you to lose weight. A keto diet is a very strict low-carb diet. You are going to consume about 20 grams or less of net carbs each day.

When you have reached your weight loss goals, you can begin to increase your carb intake. This needs to be done slowly, so you don't gain the weight back.

Basics

This is a great diet; there is a right and wrong way to do it. You have to begin this diet the right way, so you get faster and better results.

On paper, the keto diet is fairly simple: you eat low carbs and high fat. This doesn't tell you what you can and can't eat. There is a complete list of foods that are fine to eat along with foods that are restricted later in the book, but here is a basic list of what you can have:

- Meats including organ meats

- Heavy fats like butter, lard, bacon fat, ghee, olive oil, coconut oil, and tallow

- Fish and seafood

- Eggs

- Certain berries such as raspberries, blueberries, and strawberries

- Vegetables that aren't starchy. You are going to want to eat all the leafy greens you can.

This means that the food you eat on a typical day might look like:

- Breakfast: eggs and bacon

- Lunch: a cup of bone broth and chicken salad

- Dinner: vegetables along with a steak and even a dessert that is ketogenic-friendly.

Some people can't go through their day without having a snack. This is fine as long as you stick with broth, cheese sticks, nuts, celery sticks, and meat sticks. You need to watch the snacks. You will have to add it into your total macros for the day.

The keto diet is easy to personalize. You have the ability to experiment and see what is going to work best for you. Some people find they need more fats in their diet while others will be able to eat more carbs. Some people even try intermittent fasting.

Many people that intermittent fast will skip breakfast and will eat their first meal at about one in the afternoon. This will up your ketosis power.

Macros

Macros have been mentioned before, and you might be wondering what they are. Macros are short for macronutrients when talking about the ketogenic diet.

Macros are parts of the food that give you fuel and energy. These are protein, carbohydrates, and fats. These are what gives you your dietary calories. It's important that you totally understand what macros are if you want to succeed with this diet. These have to be in the correct balance for you to remain in ketosis.

Carbs are the only macros that you don't have to eat to be able to live. There are essential amino acids and fatty acids that are building blocks for fats and proteins, but carbohydrates aren't essential.

Carbs are made up of two things' sugars and starches. Fiber is looked at as a carb, but with the keto diet, it doesn't get counted into your total carb intake. Fiber isn't counted because your body doesn't digest fiber, so it doesn't affect your blood sugar.

When you look at a nutrition label on a food, you need to look at the total carb amount and then look at the fiber. You will need to subtract the total about of fiber from the total amount of carbs. This gives you your net carb amount.

Total carbs – fiber = net carbs

What this means is that net carbs only count the sugars and starches in the carbohydrates. What you are trying to figure your macros for your meals, you only use the net carbs. You don't have to use the total number of carbs.

In order to succeed, you need to find foods that are low in carbohydrates naturally and the ones that aren't. Not all of them are obvious. It is obvious that potatoes are high in carbs, but did you know that bananas are also high in carbs?

For people who are just beginning the keto diet, they should try to consume about 20 grams of net carbs every day.

Protein is important for the body since it helps keep lean muscle mass, a source of energy when carbs aren't available, makes hormones and enzymes, immune function, growth, and tissue repair. Protein has an important role in the body's biological process. Proteins are called the building blocks of a healthy body.

When we consume proteins, they get broken down into amino acids. Nine of these aren't able to be produced by the body. This is why we need to get these essential amino acids from the foods we eat. These nine essential amino acids are phenylalanine, valine, histidine, tryptophan, isoleucine, threonine, leucine, methionine, and lysine. Where there's a deficiency in protein or any of these amino acids, it could cause malnutrition, kwashiorkor, or many other health problems.

When you are following a ketogenic diet, you need to make sure you eat enough protein to preserve your lean body mass. The amount you consume depends on the amount of lean body mass you have right now. Here is a guideline:

- 0.7 to 0.8 grams of protein per pound of muscle to help preserve your muscle mass.

- 0.8 to 1.2 grams of protein per pound of muscle to increase your muscle mass.

You don't want to ever lose body mass. You need to aim to preserve or gain. Many people only focus on losing weight, but a lot of the time, losing weight means losing muscle along with the fat. Your goal should be to lose fat and save your muscle. This is important for you to keep good metabolism.

The main thing to remember is not to go crazy when you eat protein while doing keto. Too much might end up putting stress on your kidneys, and this can affect ketosis. Aim to keep your macros in the above ranges.

Take a look at this example:

Let's say you weigh 160 pounds and you have a body fat percentage of 30 percent. This would mean you have about 48 pounds of body fat. Now you are going to subtract your body fat from your total weight. This gives you your lean body mass. For this example, it would be 112 pounds.

In order to figure out the amount of protein you need to eat, you need to take your lean body mass number and multiply by the ratio from earlier. For this example, you need to consume 89.6 grams of protein every day to preserve your muscle mass. It would look like this:

112 pounds muscle X .8 grams of protein = 89.6 grams

The last macro is fats. We need to consume a decent amount of fat to maintain cell membranes, provide cushioning for protecting the organs, absorbing specific vitamins, growth, energy, and development. These fats also help you feel fuller longer.

Dietary fats get broken down into fatty acids and glycerol. Our bodies can't synthesize two types of fatty acids, so we have to include them in our diets. These fatty acids are linolenic acid and linoleic acid.

These fats are sating, so it is perfect for anyone who is looking to help fight hunger pangs. Now all you have to do is figure out the amount of fat you need to eat. If your carbs are at the lowest possible, you know how much protein you need to consume, the rest of your dietary needs will have to be met with fat.

To maintain your weight, you need to eat enough calories from fat to support your normal expenditure. If you want to burn fat, then you need to eat in the deficit.

You have been given a lot of information to help you find your macros. There are easier ways to figure this out. There are many online calculators to help you figure out these numbers without getting a headache. If you would like to use an online calculator, check out the website Ketogains. Theirs works great.

If you would like to see how figuring out for yourself will work, let's continue to use the 160-pound example from earlier. We're going to assume this person is a female, stands 5' 4", in her late 20s and sits behind a desk all day. This means she is mostly sedentary.

Let's put her information into a calculator:

Base metabolic rate is 1467 kcal.

Daily energy expenditure would be 1614 kcal.

She is going to need to eat about 90 grams of protein, 20 grams of net carbs, and 86 grams of fat. Her intake is made up of 72 percent fat, 23 percent protein, and five percent carbs.

Now that you know what macros are and the way to figure your numbers, you are on your way to beginning the ketogenic diet.

Why Try Keto?

When you are on a ketogenic diet, your body gets good at burning stored fat for its fuel. This is wonderful for many reasons. One of them is the fact that fat contains more calories than most carbs, so you can eat less food each day. Your body will easily burn the stored fat, and this results in more weight that is lost. Using fat as fuel will provide constant levels of energy. It won't spike your blood sugar, and this means you won't experience the lows and high when eating carbs. Having constant levels of energy throughout your day means you will get more done and won't feel tired when doing it.

In addition to these benefits, following a keto diet can:

- Improves brain function

- Improves HDL (good) levels and LDL (bad) cholesterol

- Reduces blood pressure

- Reduces triglycerides

- Reduces insulin resistance and blood sugar. This can reverse prediabetes and type 2 diabetes.

- Results in loss of more body fat.

There are many different things that could happen when following a keto diet. Let's talk about some.

Helps your brain focus

A ketogenic diet helps increase your clarity, memory, cognition, fewer migraines, and seizure control. The first use of this diet was in the 1920s at the Mayo Clinic to help children who had epilepsy. The exact reason behind the prevention of seizures while doing a keto diet is still unknown, but scientist thinks it is because it causes more stability in the neurons and up-regulation of mitochondrial enzymes and brain mitochondria.

Close to this, there has been some attention given to this diet and how it affects Alzheimer's disease. Researchers found there was improved memory and increased cognition in adults who had problems in these areas. More research has found improvement with every stage of dementia. Ketosis can help fight Parkinson's disease.

For the larger audience of keto followers, there have been fewer side effects and less frequent migraines, along with better mental clarity and focus. This is because of the more stable blood sugar and the change of chemistry in the brain that helps with memory and cognition.

Cancer Fighter

Dom D'Agostino's lab figured out that ketone supplementation was able to decrease the viability of tumor cells and helped to prolong the life of mince that had metastatic cancer. Cancer cell metabolism works abnormally when compared to healthy cells. These get increased through consuming glucose because of genetic mutations and mitochondrial dysfunction. Some studies show that unlike healthy tissues, cancer cells can't use ketone bodies for energy. Ketones also inhibit the proliferation and viability of tumor cells.

This isn't saying that if you have cancer, you should stop your normal treatments. You should always follow your doctor's advice.

Prevents Heart Disease

Following a keto diet could help lower blood pressure and triglycerides along with improving cholesterol. This happens because this diet keeps blood glucose low and stable. This might sound counterintuitive that eating fats will help you lower your triglycerides; it has been proven that eating too many carbs is the main reason behind high triglyceride levels.

When talking about LDL and HDL, the keto diet can help up HDL levels. This is the good cholesterol. It can also help to improve LDL profiles.

Decreases Inflammation

In an article in Nature Medicine, it was found that the mechanism behind what has been believed for decades: a keto diet is anti-inflammatory and could help with many other issues.

Research has found that these might be connected to "BHB-mediate inhibition of the NLRP3 inflammasome."

This basically says that inflammatory diseases can be suppressed by BHB. This is a ketone that is produced by following a ketogenic diet. This has helped other problems like arthritis, eczema, IBS, acne, psoriasis, and other inflammatory diseases that have prompted more research.

Improves Energy and Sleep

By the time people reach day four or five on the diet, many will report an increase in energy and fewer carb cravings. The main reason for this is stable insulin levels and a readily available energy source for the body tissues and brain.

It still isn't understood why it improves sleep. Studies have shown that the ketogenic diet helps with sleep because it decreases REM and increases slow-wave sleep patterns. The exact reason why is unclear. It has something to do with the complex biochemical shift involved with the brain using ketones for energy when combined with the body burning fat.

Stable Uric Acid Levels

The main cause of kidney stones and gout is elevated levels of uric acid, calcium, phosphorus, and oxalate. This is due to the combination of consuming things with many purines and alcohol, obesity, sugar consumption, unlucky genetics, and dehydration.

There is a caveat; a ketogenic diet will temporarily raise your uric acid levels, especially if you let yourself get dehydrated. With time, the levels will go back down.

Assists Gastrointestinal and Gallbladder Health

This means you will have less gas and bloating, improved digestion, less heartburn and acid reflux, and less risk of gallstones.

It is known that sugary foods, nightshades such as potatoes and tomatoes, and grain-based foods can increase the chances of a person getting acid reflux and heartburn.

It shouldn't surprise you to learn that eating fewer carbs can improve these symptoms and confront the problems of bacterial issues, inflammation, and autoimmune responses.

A ketogenic diet will rapidly and reproducibly alter our gut microbiome. Dr. Eric Westman explains how many problems are reduced or removed because of these microbiome changes.

Research has found that consuming carbs is one of the main causes of gallstones. When you eat enough fat while your intake of carbs is low, it will clear up gallbladders and make things run a lot more smoothly.

Assists with Women's Health

One review published in 2013 looked at evidence of the ways a keto diet could enhance fertility. Research shows that PCOS can be treated effectively by following a low-carb diet. This can help reduce or eliminate symptoms such as acne, obesity, and infrequent or prolonged periods.

Basically, when you keep your blood sugar low and stable, it will help to stabilize and equilibrate other hormone levels. This can cause other benefits on a large array of metabolic pathways that get treated with insulin, such as hunger and energy utilization.

Helps the Eyes

The largest problem many diabetics face is macular degeneration. It is known that high blood sugar could hurt people's eyesight and might lead to greater risks of cataracts. It shouldn't surprise you that when you keep your blood sugar levels low, it can improve your vision health and improve your eyes.

Help Muscle Gain and Improves Endurance

It has been found that BHB can help promote muscle gain. If you combine this with other evidence through the years, there has been an increase in the bodybuilder movement toward a keto approach to gain muscle.

Ultra-endurance athletes have turned to the keto diet, too. After the athlete has become completely fat-adapted, there is some evidence that suggests that their physical and mental performance will be improved.

Improves Obesity, Diabetes, and Metabolic Syndrome

This is the main reason why people begin a ketogenic diet. For all the reasons we've covered, a keto diet is wonderful for people who have been diagnosed with type 1 or type 2 diabetes.

It can also be effective for obesity because it helps burn fat and prevents muscle loss. It can also prevent disorders that are related to obesity. This includes all of the symptoms and risk factors are known as metabolic syndrome.

Chapter 2: Keto in Steps

Now that you know the science behind the ketogenic diet and the reasons it works, you are going to learn how to get started and how to maximize your success. Here is an easy and quick guide for you to use when starting. You can also look back over it anytime you need to in your journey when you need some guidance and support.

Clean Out the Pantry

When you have unhealthy, tempting foods in your house, it is the largest contributor to failure when beginning any diet. In order to succeed, you have to get rid of any triggers if you want to maximize your chances. If you don't have the iron will of The Rock, you have to keep addictive foods such as desserts, bread, and any other non-keto-friendly snacks in your house.

If you live with others, you need to talk about what you are doing before you just throw out everything. If there are some things that you can throw away because they don't belong to you, try to find a location that will keep them out of your sight. This will let your roommates know that you are serious about your new lifestyle. It will lead to better experiences for you at home, too. Other people love to tempt others who are trying to diet when they begin, but they usually tire out quickly.

- Grains and Starches

Throw out all the croissants, rolls, wraps, bagels, bread, flour, quinoa, oats, corn, potatoes, rice, pasta, and cereal.

- Drinks and Sugary Foods

Throw out all candy bars, milk chocolate, pastries, desserts, milk, fruit juices, fountain drinks, and refined sugars.

- Legumes

Throw away all lentils, peas, and beans. These are dense with carbs. Just a one cup serving of beans will contain more than three times the number of carbs you need in one day.

- Processed Polyunsaturated Oils and Fats

Throw out all vegetable oils and most oils that are made from seeds like corn, grapeseed, soybean, canola, safflower, and sunflower. Try to get rid of any trans fats such as margarine and shortening. Basically, anything that says "partially hydrogenated" or "hydrogenated." Coconut, avocado, extra-virgin olive, and olive oil are the only oils you need to keep on hand.

- Fruits

Throw away all fruits that are high in carbs, like apples, mangos, grapes, dates, and bananas. Make sure to throw out any dried fruits such as raisins. Fruits that have been dried contains the same amount of sugar as the regular fruit, but it is more concentrated. This makes it easy to eat too much sugar in just one small serving. Look at this comparison: one cup of raisins will have over 100 grams of carbs, while a cup of grapes will only have 15 grams of carbs.

You might be "throwing out" your unwanted foods, but this food could feed others. Don't just chuck them in the garbage; donate them to a local food pantry to help feed the homeless.

Your pantry is going to look empty after you have cleaned it out. This is because products that are meant to be stored long term are full of unhealthy additives, preservatives, and carbs. We are going to fill your refrigerator in the next step.

Let's Go Shopping

Now it is time to restock your freezer, refrigerator, and pantry with keto-friendly, delicious foods that will make you feel great, get healthy, and lose weight.

- Basics

When you have these basics on hand, you will be able to prepare keto-friendly, delicious, and healthy snacks and meals.

- o Seeds and nuts like pumpkin seeds, chia seeds, flaxseed, pine nuts, hazelnuts, walnuts, almonds, pecans, and macadamia nuts.

- o Fermented and pickled foods such as sauerkraut, kimchee, and pickles.

- o Broths like bone, beef, and chicken.

- o Low-carb condiments such as Sriracha, pesto, mustard, and mayonnaise.

- o Lime or lemon juice

- o Sweeteners like erythritol and stevia

- o Any herbs and spices your heart desires

- o Tea, coffee, and water

- Meats

Any meat is fine for this diet, including wild game, turkey, pork, lamb, beef, and chicken. It is preferred to use organic or grass-fed meats if they are readily available and you can afford them. You should and can eat the fat on the meat and the skin of the chicken.

All wild-caught seafood and fish goes well with the keto diet very well. Try to stay away from any farm-raised fish.

You can have all the eggs you would like. Use free-range or organic eggs if at all possible.

- Vegetables

You are allowed to eat all the vegetables that aren't starchy like cauliflower, Summer squash, zucchini, olives, eggplant, Brussels sprouts, garlic (in limited quantities – every clove contains one gram of carbs), tomatoes, peppers, onions, lettuce, cucumbers, mushrooms, asparagus, and broccoli.

Stay away from all kinds of potatoes, sweet potatoes, yams, corn. Avoid legumes such as peas, lentils, and beans.

- Fruits

You can have a small number of berries each day like blueberries, blackberries, raspberries, and strawberries. Lime and lemon juice are great to add flavor to meals. Avocados are full of healthy fats and are very low in carbs.

Stay away from all other fruits since they are loaded with sugars. One banana contains about 25 grams of net carbs.

- Dairy

You need to eat full-fat dairies such as unsweetened yogurt, cream cheese, cheese, heavy cream, sour cream, and butter. It isn't technically dairy, but unsweetened coconut and almond milk are great to have, too.

Stay away from skim milk, sweetened yogurt, and milk because they contain sugar. Stay away from all fat-free, low fat, or any flavored dairy products.

- Oils and Fats

Bacon fat, lard, butter, olive oil, and avocado oil are great for eating and cooking. Avocado oil has a high smoke point, which is great for searing meats and frying in a wok. A high smoke point oil means the oil won't smoke or burn until it hits 520 degrees Fahrenheit. Be sure to stay away from oils that have been labeled
"blend." These will contain small amounts of healthy oils and add in large amounts of unhealthy oils.

Setting up The Kitchen

Preparing recipes is the best part of the ketogenic diet, and it is very easy when you have the correct tools. These tools will make cooking faster and easier. Each one is worth the money, especially if you cook a lot.

- ***Food Scale***

When you are trying to hit your macro and calorie goals, a food scale is completely necessary. You will be able to measure any liquid or solid food. You will get the correct amount each time. If you use it along with an app such as "MyFitnessPal," you will have all the information you need to hit your goals. You can find food scales online for around ten to 20 dollars.

- ***Food Processor***

These little beauties are essential for your kitchen. These are great for blending or processing foods together to make shakes and sauces. Blender just won't cut it for most foods like cauliflower and other tough vegetables.

One great food processor/blender is the Nurtibullet. The container you blend with has lids and drink spouts so you can make a shake and take it with you. They are easy to clean, and this makes the entire system very convenient. You can usually find these for around $80 online.

- ***Vegetable Spiralizer***

These cute little things will turn vegetables into ribbons or noodles in just seconds. They make cooking easier and faster. Noodles have more surface area and don't take as long to cook. A spiralizer can turn zucchini into noodles. Just add some marinara or Alfredo sauce, and you will never know you are eating zucchini. These cost about $30 and can either be found online or in retail stores.

- ***Electric Hand Mixer***

If you have ever tried to beat an egg white by hand until stiff peaks form, you know how hard it can be. Electric mixers will save your arms and time, especially if you are mixing heavy ingredients. You can find good ones anywhere for around $10 to $20.

- ***Cast Iron Pans***

These have been around for hundreds of years and were one of the very first modern cooking devices. Cast iron skillets won't wear out and are healthier for you since they don't contain any chemicals. They retain heat extremely well and can be taken off the stove and put straight into the oven. They are easy to clean. Just wipe them out with a non-scratchy sponge, dry them, and rub them down with cooking oil before you put them away. This will prevent them from rusting and will help season them. You will soon have a natural nonstick surface. When you buy a new cast iron pan, most will come pre-seasoned, and this preserves the coating. You can find them in any retail store or online from between $10 and $80. It all depends on the size and brand. The lodge is the most popular brand, and it is made in the United States.

- ***Knife Sharpening Stone***

The majority of your prep time will be spent cutting foods. You will see your cutting speed skyrocketed with a set of sharp knives. It is fun to use sharp knives. Try to sharpen your knives each week to keep them in tip-top shape. Sharpening stones usually cost less than $10. They can be found in most retail stores or online.

Exercise

When you exercise more, you are going to have better health. If you follow a keto diet, you are going to lose weight quickly and improve your health. What happens when you combine the two?

It would be easy to assume that combining the two will take your health and weight loss to new levels, but the truth is a bit more complicated. With the restriction of carbs, there is a lot of change that could happen, and some of these will affect how well you exercise.

With the restricted carb intake, you are limiting your muscles from getting sugar, which is the easiest fuel source. When your muscles can't access sugar, their high-intensity function will be impaired. High intensity is any activity that lasts longer than ten seconds. The reason for this is that, after ten seconds of max effort, the muscles will produce energy from glucose through a metabolic pathway called glycolysis. Glycolysis happens rather than the process in the phosphagen system.

Fat and ketones are not good substitutes for glucose during this time. After you have been exercising for two minutes, your body will shift into a metabolic pathway that will use fat and ketones.

Basically, when you are restricting your carb intake, you deprive the cells of your muscles of sugar that they need to fuel activities for high-intensity efforts for ten seconds to two minutes. This means if you are following a keto diet, it is going to limit your performance during exercises such as:

- Playing a sport that gives you minimal breaks like soccer, rugby, and lacrosse.

- Weight lifting for more than five reps each set using a weight that is heavy enough to almost cause you to fail.

- Interval training or high-intensity circuit training

- Sprinting or swimming for more than ten seconds.

This list is not comprehensive, but it will give you an idea of the types of exercises that your body uses glycolysis for. Remember that the metabolic pathway timing varies on each individual. There are people who have the capacity to maintain performance for 30 seconds without needing any carbs at all.

It is important for you to consume the correct amount of fat and protein when exercising and doing keto.

Many health professionals, when they design a diet plan, will arrange the protein intake first. This is because protein always gets top priority as it performs many actions that carbs and fats can't. Protein will help improve satiation, has a better thermic effect, and stimulates muscle synthesis better than all the other macronutrients. If enough protein isn't consumed, you will lose muscle mass and might end up eating more calories.

If you are going to keep your exercise regimen or begin one, which you really should, you need to make sure you eat the correct amount of macros. Here are some guidelines:

- The majority of your excess calories should come from fat and not protein or carbs.

- Keep the protein intake to one gram per pound of body weight.

- Be sure your calorie intake stays around a deficit of 250 to 500 calories. This is not a top priority. Many people don't worry about calories all the much when doing a keto diet.

Now that you have to be careful and smart with eating while exercising, let's learn some exercises that are good with keto.

Keto Along with Cardio

The good thing for most of us is we aren't athletes, so adding an exercise routine won't be hard. Cardio workouts don't require you to exercise intensively to require your body to burn glycogen and sugar for you to see the results. You just have to work to bring your heart rate up and keep it there.

Because cardio is a low to moderate intensity exercise, a keto diet won't impair your performance. You might realize that you have the ability to work out for a longer time without tiring as quickly when you are in ketosis.

The intensity you need to aim for in order to get the most out of your workout is moderate intensity. When you aim for moderate-intensity physical activity, you should get your heart rate to 50 to 70 percent of your max heart rate.

In order for you to estimate your max heart rate, begin by subtracting your age from 220. If you are 50 years old, to figure out your age-related heart rate, you would take 220 and subtract 50. This gives you 170 beats per minute. This you can figure out the 50 to 70 percent levels, which would be:

- 70 percent – 170 x 0.70 = 119

- 50 percent – 170 x 0.50 = 85

This means that a 50-year-old person, in order to partake in moderate=intensity physical activity, you need to keep your heart between 85 and 119 beats per minute.

When you set out yourself to keep a ketogenic diet, your objective should be to aim for the bottom end of the range. When you have been on the diet for a couple of weeks, you will begin to see that you can maintain a higher heart rate without needing any extra carbs.

If you are new to working out and cardio, you want to stick to 50 percent of your max heart rate for around ten to 15 minutes. You can begin increasing the duration by five or so every week until you can work out for 30 to 45 minutes at 50 percent of your max heart rate. When you have managed to do this, you can start increasing your intensity level every week until you have reached 70 percent of your max heart rate.

If you aren't sure what works best for cardio workouts, here are some examples:

- Cycling

- Aerobic training classes

- Running

- Swimming

- Circuit training

- Recreational sports

- Interval training classes

You need to remember that your strength and power might become decreased during these workouts due to carb restriction. If you just want to get a good cardio workout, then it isn't important that you push yourself to the max for your strength and power.

This isn't saying that you can't increase your strength and power while on a keto diet. All you need to do to achieve this is practice mindful exercising.

Keto and Weight Lifting

You can increase power, muscle mass, and strength when following a ketogenic diet. The best thing to do is improve all these at the same time by using the same program.

It was stated earlier that without glucose, your body could only last for ten seconds with high-intensity exercises. This means if you are a weightlifter, you could improve strength and power, as well as muscle mass, by doing sets that won't last longer than ten seconds.

This means if you follow a program that requires five or more sets of five or fewer reps for every exercise, then this is great for people who follow a ketogenic diet.

Some research has found that lower reps might be helpful when talking about hypertrophy. This means that your muscles don't need you to pump out eight to 12 reps in a row to get bigger. What your muscles are looking for is the correct amount of volume. This depends on the person, and for your volume to increase every week.

This means that you can build muscles without carbs. Carbohydrates might be needed for some high-intensity work, but a bodybuilder doesn't have to eat a lot of carbs to see any results.

Exercise and Keto in Harmony

In order to mix these two things, you need to make the correct changes to your workout program and diet so that you don't cause any adverse reactions, especially if you do high-intensity workouts.

When you try to add in exercise just to improve your health, then you can experiment with things a bit more than an athlete can. In general, you need to try lifting weights and cardio training each week. Cardio needs to be done two to three times every week, and you need to lift weights two or three times every week. You don't need to try to do both of these on the same day.

Chapter 3: What to Expect

The ketogenic diet is safe and effective; there are some dangers and downsides. Before we go into the dangers, let's look at some side effects that you might experience when you finally enter ketosis.

Side Effects of Keto

Not all the side effects of keto are bad, but there are a few that can be definitely unpleasant.

1. You might feel tired or sick

You might have heard people talk about the keto flu. This is totally real. When you cut carbs and enter into ketosis, it can cause many uncomfortable symptoms like muscle aches, diarrhea, headaches, nausea, and fatigue. These side effects are caused by your body transitioning into learning to use fat as its source of energy instead of using carbs. When your body has finally adapted to this new fuel source, which will take about a week or two, you will notice that you begin to feel better.

2. You might lose weight fast, but it could come back

Ketogenic diets are popular because of the fast slim down. This is because your body releases a lot of water when your body begins using fat for energy. Your scales will go down a few pounds, and you might even look leaner.

That first drop you experience will probably only be water weight. This isn't saying you haven't burned off any fat. The problem is, while studies have shown that you are going to lose weight, they haven't figured out if it can be sustained long-term. Many people find that a strict eating plan is tough to stick with. If you go off the diet, you might gain back all the weight.

3. You might feel less hungry

Many diets are associated with feeling hungry and constantly fighting off cravings. This isn't necessarily true with the keto diet. There are many people who say they aren't as hungry and don't feel like eating all the time. Researchers aren't clear as to why this happens, but they believe that low-carb diets suppress ghrelin, which is a hormone that controls hunger.

4. You will feel very thirsty

Don't worry if you begin to feel parched when following a keto diet. You are going to be expelling a lot of water, and it is going to spike your thirst. Be sure you drink a lot of water. There isn't a set amount, but you need to drink enough so that your urine is clear to pale yellow.

5. *Your acne could clear up*

If you have always been bothered with acne, you might find that the keto diet might clear it up. This is especially true if you always ate a lot of sugar. Empty carbs are the worst for acne since they trigger inflammation. Studies have shown that curbing your carb intake might fix these problems.

6. *Not as much brain fog*

Everyone knows that carbs, especially refined ones such as sugar, white bread, and white paste, can cause your blood sugar to dip and spike. It is easy to see why eating less of them will keep your blood sugar steady. For people who are generally healthy, this means you will have a steady flow of energy, fewer cravings for sugar, and not as much brain fog.

7. *Your A-1C levels might get better*

If you have diabetes, having better control of your blood sugar might help you control you're a-1C. It might even reduce your need for insulin. This isn't saying you need to stop taking your meds. The main downside is that it could up your risk of developing diabetic ketoacidosis, which is life-threatening. This is more common in people who have type 1 diabetes. If you have type 2, you should still speak with your doctor first before beginning any diet.

8. *Low levels of energy*

This is normal while your body is adjusting to the switch in fuel sources. The good news for you is after your body gets adjusted, your energy levels will improve.

Dangers of Keto

Now that you know some of the side effects that the keto diet might cause, and you know not to worry. The negative ones will usually go away when your body has adjusted to this diet. The following are something that might happen to you on the keto diet that might not be temporary. These are extremely rare, but they might happen.

1. *Low blood sugar*

Most of the time, when you have reached ketosis, you will notice your blood sugar levels will be more stable and lower. This is why low-carb diets are effective in controlling type 2 diabetes. Monitoring your carbs has been used for some time now as a way to control blood sugar. One study found that diets low in carbs isn't any better for long-term control than other diets.

There is some anecdotal evidence that says people who are diabetic with type 2 diabetes were actually able to stop taking their medicine because they were able to stabilize their blood sugar. This is not recommended, and if you have diabetes, please talk with your doctor first.

During the first few days, while the body is adapting to change, your body is going to be in a constant struggle with itself. You will need to ease into this diet if you are diabetic. Slowly cut back on the carbs; otherwise, you might cause your blood sugar to drop too much.

2. Nutritional deficiencies

A diet that is high in fat and low in carbs will limit the types of foods that you can eat, and some complete food groups get eliminated altogether. Legumes, beans, and grains are all out along with many fruits and vegetables. Many of these foods carry nutrients, minerals, and vitamins that you can't get anywhere else. Without these foods, you might end up experiencing nutritional deficiencies.

Keto isn't a good idea for the long term since it isn't a completely balanced diet. Diets that don't allow fruits and vegetables will cause micronutrient deficiencies that could cause other consequences. It is great for short term fat loss, but it is best under the supervision of a medical professional.

3. Constipation and bowel changes

When you eliminate fruits and vegetables from your diet, you won't be getting the nutrients you need, and it could cause other problems, too. These are the fiber-rich foods that will keep you regular. Without these foods, you might find that you are beginning to have changed with your bowels. This might include difficulty with bowel movements and possible constipation.

You need to be sure your load up on low-carb, fiber-rich foods such as cabbage, broccoli, and asparagus, along with fats such as coconut oil and ghee.

4. Losing electrolytes

After you have hit ketosis, your body is going to begin dumping stores of glycogen that is found in your fat and muscles that carry extra weight. This is going to make you use the bathroom more and could lead to electrolyte loss. Electrolytes are important for proper cardiac function and regular heartbeats. This might cause you to get cardiac arrhythmia.

Try to add electrolytes through natural sources or with OTC supplements.

5. Decreased serum sodium

Normal Americans tend to consume too much salt, but when you are doing a keto diet, they might struggle to get enough. Low sodium can cause confusion, leg cramps, decreased energy, and vomiting. Be sure you add salt to every meal. Sea salt is best since it contains trace minerals.

6. Dehydration

This is more common for people that are just beginning the keto diet since ketosis flushes your body of water. To prevent dehydration, it is best to aim for 2.5 liters of water every day. This should begin as soon as you begin this diet. You don't need to wait until you feel side effects.

7. Kidney stones and kidney damage

If you don't take care of your dehydration, it might cause acute kidney injury. But, that isn't the only way you could hurt your kidneys with the ketogenic diet. Excess protein could create high nitrogen levels that increase the pressure on the kidneys. This could cause kidney stones and can damage your kidney cells.

8. Muscle loss

The longer you keep your body in ketosis, the more fat it is going to burn. The bad news is that you could lose muscle tissue, too. Yes, protein does help build muscle and is the powerhouse. Your muscles need carbs for formation and maintenance. Without carbs, the body might begin to break down your muscles.

9. Heart problems

Losing some heart muscle isn't the only risk associated with the heart that can happen while following the keto diet. If you already take medication for high blood pressure and you follow the keto diet, you might end up with abnormally low blood pressure results. If you have a heart condition, speak with your doctor before beginning the keto diet.

Chapter 4: Ketosis and Reaching It

You've read the word ketosis numerous times in this book. Let's find out exactly what it is. Ketosis is a natural state your body goes into when it becomes fueled by fat. This will happen when a person fasts or when they follow a strict low-carb diet.

There are many benefits for being in ketosis, like health, performance, and weight loss. Remember that being in ketosis can have some side effects. For people who have type 1 diabetes and other diseases, excessive ketosis can become dangerous.

When you are in ketosis, your body will produce ketones. These are small fuel molecules, and our bodies use them as alternative fuel sources when glucose is in short supply. The liver will begin converting fat into ketones that get released into the bloodstream. The body can use them just like glucose. Our brains can also use the ketones as fuel too.

Getting into Ketosis

There are two ways our bodies can reach ketosis: by fasting or following a ketogenic diet. Under either of these circumstances, when the body's limited amount of glucose gets depleted, the body will switch its fuel source to fat. Insulin, which is a fat storing hormone, will get low and the body's ability to burn fat increases. This means your body has easy access to your stored fat and is able to get rid of it.

You can consider yourself in ketosis after your body makes enough ketones to make a significant level in the blood, usually more than 0.5 mm. The fastest way for this to happen is fasting, but you can't do that forever.

This is why people follow the keto diet since it can be eaten for an indefinite amount of time.

Fuel for the Brain

Many people think you need carbs to fuel the brain. The brain will happily burn carbs when you eat them, but if carbs aren't available, it will eat ketones just as happily.

This is needed for basic survival. Because our bodies can only store carbs for one or two days, the brain would shut down after just a few days without food. Alternatively, it needs to quickly convert muscle protein into glucose, which isn't very effective, just to keep it working. This means we would waste away extremely fast. If this was how our bodies actually worked, then the human race would not have been able to survive before food became available 24/7.

Our bodies have evolved to work a lot smarter than that. Normally our bodies have stored fat that will last so we could survive for many weeks without food. Ketosis is the process that happens to make sure the brain can run on stored fat.

Ketosis versus Ketoacidosis

There are many misconceptions about ketosis. The main one is mixing ketosis with ketoacidosis. Ketoacidosis is a rare and dangerous condition that will normally happen to people who have type 1 diabetes. There are many health care professionals who mix these two words up, too. It could be because their names are similar, and there is a lack of knowledge between the differences.

Ketosis is a natural state that happens to the body, and the body is in total control of itself. Ketoacidosis is a malfunction of the body where it creates excessive amounts of ketones that the body can't regulate. This can cause things such as nausea, stomach pain, and vomiting; this is then followed by confusion and coma. This requires urgent medical treatment and might end up being fatal.

Ketoacidosis will happen when ketones reach a level of 10 millimolar or more. People who follow a ketogenic diet will normally reach a level of three millimolar or less. There are many people who struggle to reach 0.5. Long-term starvation, which happens when you have gone without food for 7 or more days, could bring the number up to six or seven. Ketoacidosis might happen at level ten, but it normally happens around 15 and above.

The difference between these two things is like drinking a glass of water versus drowning in the ocean. Both of these things deal with water, but they are nowhere near being the same thing.

If you have a properly functioning pancreas that produced insulin, which basically means you haven't been diagnosed with type 1 diabetes, it is going to be extremely hard for you to hit ketoacidosis even if you tried to. The reason for this is your body will release insulin when your body produces too many ketones, which shuts down ketone production.

Getting to Optimal Ketosis

This is the state everyone who follows the keto diet wants to get to. Once you reach optimal ketosis, your body will burn fat at the fastest speed possible. In order to get to this optimal ketosis level, you have to follow a low-carb, high-fat diet as stated above and keep your macros at the optimal level. There aren't any tricks to help you reach this level. There are some things that you can do.

Here are the different ketone levels you could have:

- Below 0.5 means you aren't in ketosis.

- Between 0.5 and 1.5 is a light level of nutritional ketosis. You will be losing weight, but it isn't in an optimal range.

- Around 1.5 to 3 is the optimal ketosis level and is the best for maximum weight loss.

- Levels over 3 aren't needed. High levels aren't going to help you one way or the other. It could harm you since it means that you aren't getting enough food.

There are many people who think they are eating a strict keto diet but end up being surprised when they measure their blood ketone levels. When they measure their blood, they end up being about 0.2 or 0.5, which is nowhere near that sweet spot.

The trick to getting past this plateau is you have to make sure you stay away from obvious sources of carbs but make sure your protein intake doesn't go higher than the fat intake. It was said before that protein won't change your glucose levels as carbs do, but if you do eat too much, especially if they exceed your fat intake, it will change your glucose. This is going to compromise your optimal ketosis level.

The secret to getting around this problem is to eat more fat. You can easily do this by adding a large dollop of herbed butter on top of your steak. This might keep you from eating too much or even eating seconds.

Drinking a cup of bulletproof coffee could also help you with hunger pangs and keep you from eating too much protein. This is easy as all you have to do is add a tablespoon of butter and a tablespoon of coconut oil to your morning coffee.

When you eat more fat, you will feel fuller. This makes sure you don't eat too much protein, and this helps you eat fewer carbs. This will help you reach an optimal level of ketosis.

How to Measure Ketosis

There are several ways to figure out if you have reached ketosis. The first way is to measure ketones in your blood. This means you will have to purchase a meter and requires you to prick your finger.

There are several reasonably priced gadgets out there that will help you do this, and it will only take a few seconds to figure out what your blood ketone level is. Many people won't go to this extreme to figure out what their ketone level is, but this is the most accurate and effective.

You need to measure your blood ketones first thing every morning and on a fasted stomach. You can follow the levels that were listed earlier in this chapter to find out if you are in ketosis.

These meters will measure the amount of BHB that is in your blood. This is the main ketone that is present when you are in ketosis. The biggest downside of using this method is you have to draw blood.

Getting a test kit costs about $30 to $40 and might cost an extra $5 for each test. This is the main reason why people who choose this test will only test once each week or only every other week.

Okay, let's say you don't want to spend more money on a blood ketone meter. Here are nine options that will help you figure out if you are in ketosis:

1. Ketones in breath and urine

If you don't like the thought of pricking your finger, you can measure blood ketones by using a breath analyzer. This will check for acetone, which is one of the three ketones that will be present in your blood when you have reached ketosis.

This lets you know when your ketone levels have hit ketosis since acetone will leave the body when you reach nutritional ketosis. Breath analyzers are very accurate but not as accurate as monitoring your blood.

Another way you can check for ketosis is to check for ketones in the urine each day using special strips. This is a cheap and quick method to use to assess what your ketone levels are each day. However these aren't extremely reliable methods.

2. Bad breath

This doesn't sound very pleasant, but many people have said that they have noticed bad breath once they have hit ketosis. This is a very common side effect. People say that their breath seems fruitier.

The reason for this is the elevated ketone levels. The main culprit is the ketone acetone that the body excretes through urine and breath. While you might not like the idea of having bad breath, it is a great way to know you are in ketosis. Many people will brush their teeth more often or chew sugar-free gum.

3. Weight loss

This is probably the most obvious way to know you are in ketosis. When you first begin a keto diet, you will lose some weight very fast, but this is normally water weight when you experience another drop in weight, which will be your fat stores. This is how you will know that you are in ketosis.

4. Better focus and energy

Many people will sometimes report feeling tired, sick or having brain fog when they begin a keto diet. This is called the keto flu, but people who follow this for a long time report increased focus and better energy. Your body needs to take time to adapt to this new diet. When you hit ketosis, your brain begins burning ketones for energy, and this might take a week or two to begin happening.

Ketones are a more potent fuel source for the brain when compared to carbs. This means it will improve your brain function and mental clarity.

5. Appetite suppression

Many people say their hunger decreases when they begin following a keto diet. The reason behind this is still being researched. However, it is thought that the reduction in hunger is due to the increase in protein and vegetable consumption along with the change in your hunger hormones. The ketones might affect the way your brain reacts to hunger.

6. Digestive issues

With all the major changes to the foods you are eating, you might experience some constipation or diarrhea when you first start this diet. This lets you know that you have almost reached ketosis. When the transition period is over, these problems should go away.

7. Short-term fatigue

When your body begins making the switch into ketosis, it could cause weakness and fatigue. This makes it hard for some people to stick with the diet. This is a normal side effect, but it lets you know you are hitting ketosis.

This crappy feeling might last for one week to one month before you fully hit ketosis, but in order to help reduce this feeling, you can take an electrolyte supplement.

8. Performance decrease

Just like the point above, fatigue could cause a slight decrease in exercise performance. This is because of the reduction in your muscle glycogen stores. This is what normally provides you with the fuel you need for your high-intensity workouts. After a week or two, your performance levels should return to normal.

9. Insomnia

The biggest issue that many keto followers have is insomnia, especially when they first begin this diet. When your carbs become drastically reduced, it could cause some problems with sleeping. But, just remember that this, too, shall pass.

There are many different symptoms and signs that will tell you if you are in ketosis, and if you are doing the right things. Ultimately, if you follow the rules for a keto diet and you stay consistent, your body will be in some form of ketosis.

If you want to know absolutely for certain if you are or aren't in ketosis, the best way to do this is by using a blood ketone monitor.

Chapter 5: What Type is Right for You

Now that you know all the positive and negative aspects of this diet, it is time to decide which diet would work best for you. Yes, there is more than one type of keto diet. To make sure that you get the most from it, you should pick the diet that will work best for your health goals and needs. Every type will work best for various types of lifestyles.

Four Kinds of Keto

There are four different types of ketogenic diets that you could follow, depending on your life goals.

Here is one example, if you lead an active lifestyle or you are an athlete who likes doing high-intensity training, there is one keto diet that will be perfect for you. If you just want to lose some fat and reach our best healthy, there is one that will be perfect for you, as well.

1. The standard ketogenic diet – fat loss and therapeutic purposes.

2. Targeted ketogenic diet – workout performance.

3. Cyclical ketogenic diet – bodybuilders and athletes.

4. High-protein ketogenic diet – high protein needs.

Every one of these diets has its own rules, and they differ in the number of net carbs you get to eat every day.

Standard Ketogenic Diet

This is the best option for beginners and anyone who wants to lose body fat, and for people who want to follow it for insulin resistance and therapeutic purposes.

You will begin eating 20 or fewer net carbs each day, and for the remainder of your diet is made up of 75 percent fats and 20 to 25 percent protein.

This is the most common ketogenic diet and is probably the best one to begin with if you haven't ever followed a keto diet before. This is the diet that is used to describe what the keto diet is and works best for most people.

The rules for the standard diet are:

- 20 grams of net carbs every day. Some resources tell you that you could actually eat up to 50 grams of carbs, but if you want to reach ketosis, you have to eat 30 or fewer grams daily.

- A decent amount of protein usually about .8 grams per pound of lean muscle mass.

- High amount of fat intake.

Targeted Ketogenic Diet

This version is for people who know their bodies extremely well when it is ketosis and people who want to have extra energy for their exercise routines.

Your net carb intake is going to be about 20 to 50 fewer grams each day, normally 30 minutes to one hour before exercising. This is great for athletes who are very active.

This type of keto diet is targeted specifically to give you energy for workouts. Targeted refers to eating just after or before your workout times. This type of keto is best for people who know their limits and want the push themselves out of ketosis. This is great when you want to maintain exercise performance and lets glycogen re-synthesis happen without interrupting ketosis.

When you follow the targeted diet, you need to eat about 20 to 50 grams of net carbs in the hour right before you begin your workout. This is the number of carbs that will make up your day.

This diet is best for people who don't need to carb load, like people who follow a cyclical ketogenic diet and for people who don't want to exert any energy that would be needed to get the most out of a cyclical diet.

The best kinds of carbs to eat for the targeted diet are high on the glycemic index since these can be easily digestible. You need to aim for foods that are high in glucose and try to avoid fructose. Fructose gives the liver the glycogen it needs instead of creating glycogen from muscles, which is what the keto diet tries to avoid.

This helps to avoid ketosis being disturbed since the carbs will be burned quickly and effectively during your workout. If you are eating the majority of your carbs close to the time of your workouts, you will need to watch for hidden carbs.

Both the targeted and cyclical diets are used for high-intensity exercise, but just because you are an athlete or lead an active lifestyle doesn't mean you have to follow either one of these keto diets.

Eating extra carbs has been recommended for active people or who perform high-intensity exercise regularly; however, there is some research that shows this isn't necessarily the case.

Cyclical Ketogenic Diet

This is the best type for athletes, bodybuilders, and people who have done a keto diet before.

For this diet, you will eat a low number of net carbs for five to six days a week. Then you will eat a higher number of carbs for the other days of the week, and these cycles just repeat. People who absolutely have to eat carbs need to follow this diet.

The cyclical diet works along the lines of intermittent fasting that is followed with the 5/2 style of fasting since it has up and down days. The cyclical diet involves eating a keto diet for the majority of the week and then followed by a day or two of eating high carbs. These days are called carb-loading days.

Carb-loading involves alternating days of a keto diet with high-carb consumption days. These high-carb days might be 24 to 48 hours long. Normally, a cyclical diet requires you to consume about 50 grams of net carbs each day during the first phases and then 150 to 200 grams of net carbs during the last phase.

Just like the targeted diet, a cyclical diet is best for people who understand their limits and can't break through their boundaries without some carb consumption.

This is best for athletes and bodybuilders who want to maximize their fat loss while building their lean muscle mass.

For advanced athletes who perform high volume and high-intensity exercises would be the biggest advantage for this keto diet. The goal of the cyclical diet is to deplete your muscle glycogen between your carb-loading, while a targeted diet has the goal of keeping your muscle glycogen at a moderate level.

High Protein Ketogenic Diet

This type of ketogenic diet is best for people who want to follow the standard diet but want or need to eat more protein.

This works pretty much exactly like the standard ketogenic diet, except you eat more grams of protein every day. This means that instead of eating 5 percent carbs, 70 percent fats, and 25 percent protein, you will be eating 5 percent carbs, 60 percent fats, and 35 percent protein. This is great for anyone who lifts weights four to six days a week.

Even though you will be eating more protein with this diet, it isn't going to be enough to cause your blood sugar level to go up and knock you out of ketosis. One large myth that circles around this diet are that if you consume too much protein, it is going to knock you out of ketosis because of gluconeogenesis.

The process of GNG is very stable. You can't cause the rate of GNG to increase even if you eat extra protein. GNG is the process of making glucose from non-carbs, but it won't work at the rate of carb metabolism.

When someone eats chocolate cake, it is going to make their blood glucose spike because of all the sugar in a very small window of time. When someone eats more protein, it isn't going to cause a spike in your blood sugar since the GNG is going to stay stable.

Muscle Maintenance

If you are worried about losing muscle mass while following the ketogenic diet, your body has mechanisms that will help with muscle growth and maintenance while following this diet.

The ketones that the liver makes for energy contains protein-sparing properties, which prevents your muscles from breaking down. This is called beta-hydroxybutyrate or BHB.

Adrenaline plays a role in preserving muscle mass while in ketosis. When you have a drop in blood sugar, your body sends out a signal to produce adrenal secretions. Researchers have found that this secretion will help regular muscle mass by adrenergic influences.

This means that when the blood glucose drops due to a decrease in the intake of carbs, your body will send a signal to the adrenal glands that tell it to release epinephrine. Muscle proteins are greatly affected by these types of influences because of their hormonal activity that inhibits muscle breakdown.

This takes us back to the high protein diet. This diet, as stated above, have you eat more protein than is normally recommended for ketosis. When you eat an adequate amount of protein, it helps you maintain muscle mass.

While it appears that you are eating low amounts of protein, remember that when your body has become keto-adapted, it is going to use ketones and fats for energy, which allows it to depend on these for fuel instead of protein.

How to Choose the Right Diet

There isn't a straight forward answer to this question. The "calories in versus calories out" rule will only work to an extent. When this is followed, it doesn't think about what you are burning, lean mass or body fat.

While it might seem simple, meaning it doesn't matter what you are eating as long as you expend more than you take in, there are still other variables that haven't been put into play.

You are going to lose weight when you eat at a calorie deficit, but some of the weight you are losing could come from muscle. Research has found that even though you are consuming 15 to 25 percent of protein while doing the keto diet, you can eat at a calorie deficit while in ketosis without burning muscle mass.

If you are a beginner, it would be best for you to begin with the standard ketogenic diet. This allows your body to adjust to the diet in the easiest and quickest way and will make the transitioning into ketosis a lot easier.

Even if you are active, an athlete, starting with the standard keto diet will help guarantee the change in metabolism so that you won't need to question whether or not you have reached ketosis.

After you have brought up your ketone levels, add in some carb-loading days might be an option for you. These carb-loading days shouldn't be used as a cheat day. You need to be careful since any of these high carb days might kick you out of ketosis, and then it might take you a week or so to get back into ketosis.

Chapter 6: Making Keto Work for You

A lot of people choose not to go on a diet because they are afraid that they won't be able to implement it in their lives. The amazing thing about a ketogenic diet is that it is not all that hard to implement, and shouldn't affect your life. To help put everybody's mind at ease about following a keto diet, we are going to look at various ways to make your life easier.

Budget

Many people will assume that following a keto diet will be expensive, but it doesn't have to be. You will be eating more fat, and this will make you feel fuller than carbs. This means that you won't be eating as much. Since you likely won't need snacks, you'll save money.

Since protein stays about the same, you won't have to buy a bunch of expensive meats. The following are some money-saving tips:

- Keep it simple. You don't have to make fancy meals. The fewer ingredients you need, the more money you will save. If all you have for breakfast is a simple omelet with water, it will cost you about $3.50, if that. A Big Mac is $5.

- Get fresh vegetables when they are in season. The rest of the time, go with frozen.

- Buying a whole chicken and cutting it apart on your own is typically cheaper. You can also use the bones to make your own bone broth.

- Make sure you take notice of deals that your grocery store has and stock up when things go on sale, especially if you use them a lot.

It's best if you take the time to plan out your shopping list and meals. This will keep you organized. You will make you less likely to buy things that you don't need. Having a shopping list is the best way to keep unnecessary spending at bay.

When you are shopping, here are a few things that you can do to save money:

- Buy block cheese in bulk, and stick to regular cheeses. You can shred your own cheese.

- You can make your own coleslaw, so don't be packaged.

- Purchase simple meats instead of specialty. Cooked meats make a great quick meal but go with things that are less exotic.

- You don't have to worry about kale because it is one of the more expensive greens. You can pick other greens that are cheaper and just as nutritious.

- Avoid nuts as much as you can because they do add up.

- Pick almond meal instead of almond flour. It's cheaper and works just like almond flour. You could also make your own out of almonds.

- Don't buy avocados when not in season.

- Purchase canned or frozen fish instead of fresh, especially if you like salmon.

Get the best quality of food that fits into your budget. Just because everybody tells you that you have to eat organic doesn't mean you have to listen to them. If something doesn't fit into your budget, don't get it. The most important thing is for you to cook your own meals. They are going to be healthier whether you used organic or not.

When you are choosing meats, go with the cheaper cuts. Never forget to check out those yellow stickers; they normally have a good deal. Cooking meals at home are going to be cheaper than trying to find keto at restaurants.

Traveling

The most important thing for any diet to be sustainable is being able to eat when not at home. The key to sticking to keto when traveling is to plan things out. Keep the following in mind.

- Be aware of your macros

Before you head out on vacation, you need to make sure that you know your macros. Have them memorized, or have a keto app so that you can track them.

- Evaluate your trip

The next thing you need to do is figure out how long your trip is going to be. If it is only overnight, that will be pretty easy to plan for. A couple of frozen meals, a cooler, and a microwave are all you need. If it is going to be weeklong, that can create some complications. Knowing what you are getting ready to face, though, will help.

After you know the length of the trip and where you are going, you can look at what resources you will have when you arrive. If you can, finding a hotel room with a kitchen is a great idea. Airbnb is a great idea. Finding places that allow you to cook more will improve your flexibility. At the very least, try to find a place that has a full-size fridge and freezer. If you are staying with family or friends, then you have less to worry about.

Knowing how you are traveling is the last thing to worry about. If you are driving, things will be a bit more flexible than if you are on a plane. TSA restrictions will likely prevent you from bringing certain foods because they have to be repacked and weigh less than three ounces.

- Food choices

Now you need to think about the foods that you can take with you. Foods that don't have to be refrigerated are great. Things like canned chicken and fish and beef jerky are great. Olives and canned protein shakes are perfect too. All of the regular snack foods like nuts, string cheese, and pepperoni should definitely be packed. If you enjoy eggs, try to hard-boil some.

When it comes to perishables, you will want to buy them once you arrive unless your vacation spot is fairly close to home. You can try packing a cooler with ice to keep things fresh if you want.

Once you arrive, buy some cheese and meats. If you want, you can make all of your meals ahead of time and freeze them before your trip. Pack them up in a cooler and then set them out the morning you want to eat them.

- Restaurants

You can find fast food places and other restaurants that offer low-carb options. You can ask places to wrap your burger in lettuce and leave off the bun. Sticking with steak or fish is great. Avoid fries as the side, as well as rice and beans. Try going for a salad or veggies. If there is a Chipotle nearby, then you can get a bowl without the rice and beans and fill it up with meat, sour cream, cheese, and guacamole.

Travelling doesn't mean if you have to quit eating right. There are a lot of ways to work around these things.

Keto While Dining Out

There will come a time when you are faced with having to eat out on keto. You don't want to live the rest of your life, afraid to go out with your friends and family. Here are some tips to help.

- *Avoid the starch*

Turn down bread, don't order pasta or potatoes, and stay away from rice. Don't allow temptations to touch your plate, so order things without starches. The majority of restaurants will allow you to substitute the starchy side for extra vegetables or a salad. If you are in the mood for a burger or sandwich, see if they are willing to wrap it in lettuce instead. If they don't let you make a substitution, then eliminate the item.

If you do get your plate and there is a starch on it, look at your options. If you believe you can keep it on your plate and be tempted not to touch it, then keep it there. If you don't think you can handle it, ask the water to get rid of the starch. If you are at a casual place, you can just throw it out on your own.

- **Add some healthy fats**

Restaurants tend to serve low-fat meals, which makes it hard to feel full without carbs. This can be fixed. Ask them for extra butter that you can add to your veggies or meat. Get a vinaigrette dressing. A seasoned keto dieter will have a small bottle of olive oil with them since restaurants tend to use cheap vegetable oils that have a lot of omega 6 fats.

- **Pay attention to sauces and condiments**

Sauces like Béarnaise are mainly fats. Ketchup will normally be mostly carbs, and gravies could go either way. If you aren't sure, ask the waiter what's in them so that you don't end up eating hidden carbs. You can also ask to have the sauce on the side so that you can make your own decision on how much.

- **Be wise on drinks**

The best things to pick are water, sparkling water, coffee, or unsweetened tea. If you want alcohol, pick a dry wine, champagne, or spirits. Spirits should be mixed only with club soda or kept straight.

- **Dessert**

If you're not hungry, have a cup of coffee or tea while the others have dessert. If you want dessert, go for a cheese plate or berries with whipped cream.

- **Buffets**

This can become a problem. Create some ground rules for yourself. Stay away from starches and grains and go for fats, protein, and vegetables. Pick a small plate. You can go back for seconds if you know you are still hungry. Take your time when you eat. Talk with the people you are with and sip on your drink to eat more slowly.

You're Not a Cook

Maybe you tend to come home late, or you just don't like cooking. You unexpectedly find you don't have the stuff to make something keto. How can you work around these problems?

1. Have something to drink

If you are just trying to wait until your next planned meal, have tea or coffee loaded with some healthy fats to help curb your appetite.

2. Have low-carb snacks

You don't have to cook. You can make an appetizer plate for your dinner full of healthy, keto snacks.

3. Have leftovers

When you do cook, make enough so that you can have leftovers on those days when you don't want to cook.

4. Use a slow cooker

This is perfect if you do work late. You can prep this in the morning, and it will be ready for you when you get home.

Holidays

Holidays are the worst for diets, but if you don't want to mess up your new good habit, a little planning can go a long way. The most important thing is not to be the annoying dieter who tries to keep others from eating what they want. Keep yourself composed. You eat what you want to eat, and they can have what they want.

If you are visiting family and you want to find out what is normally in certain dishes that you didn't fix, there's an app for that. This will help you to make smart decisions. If you tend to find yourself coveting that cake on the dessert table, make sure you volunteer to take the dessert. Make a dessert or two that you know that you can have without any fear.

It also helps to try to avoid debating with others. You are seeing family you likely don't see very often, and they may give you a hard time for your new eating style. On the other hand, you may feel like bragging. It's best, though, not to engage. You're not there to fix the way your family eats. Look out for yourself.

The last thing, it is the holidays, and if you slip, it is not the end of the world. If you don't want to break your mom or grandma's heart by turning down their signature dish, then eat some of it. Get a little bit and enjoy it. You can have a few of the goodies, just know your limits and don't go hog wild. Enjoy yourself and listen to your body. You don't have to be super strict all the time. Just make sure you don't let yourself fall completely off the wagon.

Chapter 7: What You Should and Shouldn't Eat

You know the basics of a ketogenic diet, and you know, pretty much, what you should and shouldn't do. Now is the time to find out exactly what foods you can and can't eat while on a ketogenic diet.

What You Shouldn't Eat

We'll start with everything that you need to cut out of your diet, or at least greatly reduced.

- Sugar – this is the biggest no-no. You have to get rid of vitamin water, sports drinks, fruit juices, and soft drinks. Also:

    o Breakfast cereals

    o Frozen treats

    o Donuts

    o Chocolate bars

    o Cookies

    o Cakes

    o Candy

    o Sweets

- Beer – this is basically liquid bread.

- Fruit

- Margarine – you want to use real butter, not fake butter.

- Pre-packaged low-carb foods – make sure you read the label before you buy these. Even Atkins products aren't all low-carb.

- Starch:

    o Muesli

    o Porridge

    o Potato chips

- o French fries
- o Sweet potatoes
- o Potatoes
- o Rice
- o Pasta
- o Bread
- o Lentils
- o Beans

Foods You Should Eat

Now that you know what you need to avoid, let's look at everything that you get to enjoy while on a ketogenic diet.

- Dark chocolate – aim for finding chocolate that has a cocoa amount of more than 70%. 85% is the ideal cocoa amount.

- Alcohol – if you must have alcohol, try dry wine, vodka, brandy, whiskey, and anything that doesn't have sugar added.

- Water – this is a must-have.

- Coffee – make sure you don't add anything except for butter or coconut oil.

- Tea – any tea you would like, just don't add sugar.

- Bone broth – this can help add electrolytes and nutrients.

- Berries – these are good in moderation. These include raspberries, blackberries, strawberries, and blueberries.

- High-fat dairy – the more fat, the better. Butter is the best, and high-fat cheeses are good. High-fat yogurts should be consumed in moderation. Regular milk has too much sugar, so avoid it.

- Nuts – you can have these in moderation. The best are macadamia, Brazil, and pecans.

- Above ground vegetables – pick vegetables that are grown above the ground, especially green vegetables. The best are:

  - o Cauliflower

- Cabbage

- Avocado

- Broccoli

- Zucchini

- Spinach

- Asparagus

- Kale

- Green beans

- Brussels sprouts

- Seafood and fish – these are all great options, especially salmon, which is high in fat.

- Eggs – these are great because you can fix them in all different ways.

- High-fat sauces – a lot of the fat you eat should come from natural sources like eggs, fish, and meat, but you can also use fats for cooking, such as coconut oil and butter.

- Meats – all unprocessed meats are low in carbs and great for keto. The best are grass-fed and organic meats. You have to remember that you're supposed to eat high in fats and not proteins, so don't go crazy. Watch out for processed meats like meatballs, sausages, and cold cuts. They sometimes have added carbs.

Chapter 8: Is It Right for You

While the keto diet is a great and effective tool for weight loss, it may not be the right diet for you. Chances are, before reading this book, you had heard about the keto diet and decided that it was just another fad that won't last, but it has been followed for over 100 years. You are already aware of all the health benefits that the diet brings, and all of this is due to ketosis. But, it is this ketone adaptation that can cause some safety problems that you need to keep in mind. This is why I have provided you with this chapter because it may not be a good idea for everybody. The following are some situations where a ketogenic diet may be dangerous. While you may still be able to follow it, you will want to exercise caution and do so under a doctor's supervision.

Pregnant or Nursing

There aren't a lot of studies done on the effects of a keto diet on a pregnant woman. Some studies, though, have found that some side effects could include weight loss, anemia, nutrient deficiency, hormonal changes, dehydration, inadequate growth in the fetus, and constipation.

Prolong ketosis while pregnant could end up causing developmental problems for the baby that can end up affecting the development of their brain and increases the risk of defects, such as spina bifida. Due to the problems that it could cause the baby, doctors do not recommend this diet for pregnant women.

Much like with a pregnant woman, there aren't too many studies about what keto can do to a nursing woman. Most women who are nursing or pregnant often need more protein and fiber than other women. The increased fiber helps to support the development and growth of the fetus, helps with their digestion, and provides both mom and baby with the vitamins and minerals they need.

Since we don't know for certain the exact results of a ketogenic diet on nursing women, it is best to follow a moderate carb intake that is safe for the mother and the baby.

Medication-Caused Hypoglycemia

The most common hypoglycemia-causing medications are:

- Insulin

- Sulphonylureas, such as glibenclamide, tolbutamide, gliclazide, glipizide, and glimepiride.

- Glinides, such as nateglinide or repaglinide.

All of these medications are made to help increase insulin in the body. This will then lower a person's blood sugar levels. If you are following a ketogenic diet while on these medications, it could increase your odds of developing hypoglycemia. It is important that you speak to your doctor so that both of you can work together to prevent you from developing hypoglycemia before you start keto.

Making sure that you take regular blood glucose tests will give you the ability to spot and avoid developing hypoglycemia. You will have to perform tests more often than normal while your body works to adjust to the change of carbohydrate intake.

Diabetes or Blood Sugar Problems

There are plenty of people who suffer from diabetes or blood sugar problems that can follow a keto diet without any problems. There are some, however, who try to follow a keto diet and will suffer from low blood sugar when they first start. This can turn out to be dangerous if you are unable to stabilize your blood sugar while on diabetes medications.

There is a lot of evidence that shows that diabetes can be slowed or prevents through a healthy diet and exercise. To be on the safe side, people who have a history of hypoglycemia, prediabetes, or diabetes should consult with their doctor before they begin a ketogenic diet.

Changes in your diet and weight loss could mean that you need to change your diabetes medication dosage. Only your doctor can make these. You should never change your medication without talking with your doctor first.

On Other Medications

The majority of medications won't cause significant risk, but you should still do some research and speak with your doctor to make sure there won't be any problems. Your doctor will know if they need to change the dosage. Blood pressure medications could end up needing to be regulated more by your physician because a keto diet could cause your blood pressure to drop too low.

Underweight or Nutrient Deficient

The ketogenic diet is meant as a way to lose weight, and weight loss tends to happen quickly. If you are currently underweight, have vitamin or mineral deficiencies due to not eating right, or have suffered from past eating disorders, this is not the right diet for you. If your BMI is in the underweight range and you want to follow a keto diet to improve your blood sugar levels, and you don't want to lose weight, please talk to your doctor to help you to modify the diet to ensure that your weight isn't affected.

If you tend to lose weight easily, a diet with more complex carbs along with plenty of healthy fats and proteins is the best thing. If you have ever undergone gastric bypass surgery, the ketogenic diet may be dangerous because of the risk of nutrient deficiencies that can happen from not consuming enough calories.

Children

While there have been many children suffering from epileptic seizures who have been treated with a ketogenic diet, they were under medical supervision. There are many different things that you need to remember before starting a ketogenic diet for a child is to make sure that the macronutrients are balanced and appropriate for them. You absolutely must speak with a doctor or dietitian before you allow your child to start a keto diet.

Kidney Disease or Stones

The keto diet has the ability to cause kidney stones. If you already have a history of kidney disease, it probably isn't worth it to try and follow a ketogenic diet. If you have a history of any type of kidney disease, you have to talk with your doctor before you start this type of diet. Your doctor will need to keep an eye on your creatinine/calcium ratio to make sure that you aren't suffering from complications like nephrolithiasis, which is very dangerous calcium levels in your kidneys.

Gallstones or Gall Bladder Removal

People who suffer from gallstones are often told to stay away from fat, but that isn't necessarily the case anymore. The NHS says that a low-fat diet can cause gallstone growth. If you already suffer from gallstones, consuming more fat could cause more pain. If you are interested in a ketogenic diet, you may want to slowly start the diet or wait until your gallstones have been removed.

A study in 2014 found that high-fat diets could prevent the formation of gallstones, which could be another long-term benefit of this diet. The gall bladder has bile in it that will help your body to break down fats, so it may not seem like a smart idea to follow a high-fat diet like a ketogenic diet. There are plenty of people, though, that have had their gall bladder removed that have successfully followed the diet without any adverse effects.

Enzyme Deficiency or Defect

These are both very rare problems, but there are two big contraindications of the ketogenic diet called pyruvate carboxylase and porphyria deficiency. These are both caused by issues with the production of lipid and heme metabolism. Heme is part of the hemoglobin that carries oxygen out of the lungs and into other areas of your body.

People who suffer from these disorders will also suffer from deficiencies with some enzymes that make it hard for them to metabolize large amounts of fatty acids. They are then transported to the cell's mitochondria to make energy. If you follow this type of diet and suffer from these deficiencies or other types of beta oxidations defects, it can create dangerous complications like irregular heartbeats, nervous system deterioration, and mental changes.

Free fatty acids will build up, but the body won't be able to sue them for energy, and this is why it becomes dangerous. People who have pyruvate carboxylase and porphyria deficiency need a good supply of glucose to provide their organs with energy. If there is no glucose present because of this diet, some life-threatening problems can occur. This is known as a catabolic crisis. To avoid these problems, if you have a family history of mitochondrial disorders or you think you may have these conditions, you need to have a doctor test you before even thinking about starting a ketogenic diet.

Chapter 9: Lose 21 Pounds in 21 Days

Now has come the time for your kick-start to your ketogenic diet. We will look at each week individually as well as the meal prep journey that you will need to take. The recipes for these first 21-days will also be in this chapter as well. You can continue to use the recipes after the initial 21-day diet.

It may look as if there are not enough meals here for an entire week, but the idea here is to make meal prep easy and simple. This means that you won't have to cook for every single meal, making it easier to stick with the diet. While you will be eating the same meals a few times a week, you have the ability to alternate the days you eat them so that you don't have to eat the same things two days in a row. This will keep things from getting boring.

Each meal has a standard serving size. However, you are allowed to adjust this serving to be more or less depending on what your daily macro needs are.

There is no set menu with this; you can pick and choose what you want to have for breakfast, lunch, and dinner every day. The snacks are there if you need them. You don't have to eat a snack if you don't feel like you need one. However, having them on hand is always good. Just as an example, you could have:

- Monday

    o Roasted Avocado and Egg – Breakfast

    o Cesar Salad – Lunch

    o Burrito Bowl – Dinner

    o Buttercream Fat Bomb – Dessert

- Tuesday

    o Bacon, Eggs, and Tomatoes – Breakfast

    o Fresh Tomato and Sardine Salad – Lunch

    o Deviled Egg – Snack

    o Salami Basil Pizza – Dinner

Ultimately, what you eat each day is up to you.

Week One

Breakfast:
Bacon, Eggs, and Tomatoes

Roasted Avocado and Egg

Lunch:
Fresh Tomato and Sardine Salad

Cesar Salad

Dinner:
Burrito Bowls

Thai Shrimp Curry Noodles

Salami Basil Pizza

Snacks:
Bacon Deviled Eggs

Buttercream Fat Bombs

Pistachio Almond Fat Bombs

Roasted Avocado and Egg

This dish isn't the best dish to try and cook in advance. However, all of the ingredients can be prepped at the start of the week so that you will only have to put it together, which takes about three minutes, and then cook it for 15 minutes.

The toppings and measurements for them are optional, so the nutritional information is only for the egg and avocado. One standard serving has 465 calories, 3 g net carbs, 39 g fat, and 17 g protein.

What you need:

Favorite cheese

Pepper

Salt

Cilantro

Chopped chives

Sliced ham

Eggs, 2

Avocado, 1

What you do:

1. Start by placing your oven at 40 and prepare a glass pan.

2. Slice the avocado in half and take out the pit. Scrape out a small amount of flesh to make the hole big enough for an egg.

3. Put the avocado halves in the pan and crack an egg into the middle of each, and then add on your toppings of choice.

4. Let your avocados bake for 15 minutes, or until the yolk is set to your desired consistency. Top with cilantro and chives if you want.

Bacon, Eggs, and Tomatoes

The bacon and tomatoes can be cooked ahead of time. They can be reheated as you cook your eggs. This recipe makes only one serving and contains 380 calories, 7 g net carbs, 27 g fat, 21 g protein.

What you need:

Pepper

Salt

Roma tomatoes, 2

Bacon fat, 2 tsp.

Bacon, 2 strips

Eggs, 2

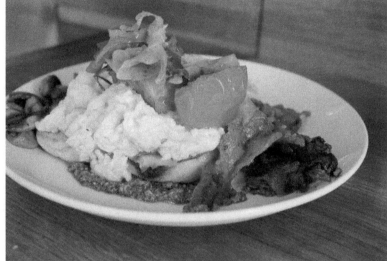

What you do:

1. On the day that you prep your meals, set your oven to 400. Place aluminum foil on a baking sheet and top with a wire cooling rack. Assemble another pan, a small glass one.

2. Put the bacon strips on the cooling rack and back for 15 to 20 minutes until crispy. Pour the extra fat into a glass jar so that you can use it later.

3. At the same time as you cook your bacon, roast your tomatoes in the glass pan. First, you need to wash and dry the tomatoes and let them roast for 25 to 30 minutes.

4. Keep the bacon and tomatoes stored in the fridge until the morning that you plan on having this for breakfast. You can reheat them in the microwave or skillet and add some pepper and salt to the tomatoes.

5. Cook your eggs the morning of in any fashion that you desire using some of the reserved bacon fat. Season and serve alongside the tomatoes and bacon.

Cesar Salad

You will need mason jars for this. They allow you to assemble the salads on your prep day, and you won't have to worry about the lettuce becoming soggy. One serving contains 626 calories, 50 g fat, 7 g net carbs, and 35 g protein.

What you need:

Pepper

Salt

Onion powder

Garlic powder

Primal Kitchen's Cesar dressing, 2 tbsp.

Parmesan cheese, 4 tbsp.

Bone-in chicken thighs, 2

Romaine lettuce, 2 servings

What you do:

1. All of this will be done on your prep day. The only thing you have to do on the day that you eat it is to shake the salad in the jar and enjoy.

2. Start by placing your oven on 375. In a glass pan, place the chicken thighs in it and top with some seasonings. Allow them to roast for 25 to 35 minutes or until they are fully cooked, and it reaches 165.

3. If you didn't by pre-washed and torn lettuce, you would need to wash, tear, and dry your lettuce.

4. Once the chicken is cooked and cooled, debone and slice it up, keeping the skin on.

5. Divide the ingredients into two portions.

6. Put the dressing at the bottom of two quart-sized mason jars, add in the cheese, the chicken, and then top with the lettuce. This order is very important because it will keep your lettuce crunchy.

Tomato and Sardine Salad

This recipe makes three servings and has 419 calories, 7 g net carbs, 31 g fat, and 27 g protein.

What you need:

Apple cider vinegar, 1 tbsp.

Dijon mustard, 2 tsp.

Celery, 2 ribs

Olive oil, 1 tbsp.

Blue cheese, .25 c

Chopped walnuts, .33 c

Heirloom tomatoes, 1.5 lbs.

Herbes de Provence

Salt

Drained capers, 2 tbsp.

Canned sardines, boneless and skinless in olive oil, 3 cans

What you do:

1. To prep the sardines, turn your broil on and open up the cans. Top them with a tablespoon of capers, herbs de Provence, and salt.

2. Cook in the oven until they are hot. The oil should be bubbling. This will take three to five minutes.

3. Wash and slice the tomatoes into bite-sized pieces.

4. Slice the celery. Toast the walnuts in a pan until fragrant. The nuts can burn quickly, so make sure you watch them. This will take around a minute.

5. Add the seasonings, olive oil, mustard, and vinegar in a bowl and whisk together.

6. Layer the salad in quart-sized mason jars. Place the vinaigrette on the bottom then add the walnuts, blue cheese, celery, tomatoes, and sardines.

7. You can serve it in the jar or pour it out on a plate when you are ready to eat.

Thai Shrimp Curry Noodles

The shrimp can be replaced with chicken if you have an allergy or if you don't like shrimp. This makes four servings, and one serving has 199 calories, 10 g net carbs, 12 g fat, and 12 g protein.

What you need:

Butternut squash "noodles" or spaghetti squash, 2 c

Salt, 2 tsp.

Thai red curry paste, 1 tbsp.

Sliced mushrooms, 8 oz.

Diced onion, 1 medium

Canned full-fat coconut milk, .5 c

Deveined large shrimp with tails removed, 10 oz.

What you do:

1. If using spaghetti squash, place the whole squash in a 9 x 13 pan with a cup or so of water. Roast at 375 for a few hours, or until you can pierce it easily with a knife. Once it is cooled, slice in half to remove the seeds, and then use a fork to flake the meat out of the inside. It will look like noodles.

2. If using butternut squash, you can spiralize your own noodles, or you can buy pre-spiralized butternut squash noodles in the produce department. Depending on where you shop, you may have a hard time finding pre-spiralized. Toss them in olive oil and salt, and roast them at 375 for around 15 to 20 minutes, or until tender.

3. Place the mushrooms and onions in a pot with the olive oil and sauté for around ten minutes.

4. Mix in the salt, red curry paste, and coconut milk. Bring everything up to a simmer.

5. Once it is simmering, add in the shrimp, cover the pot, and allow it to cook until the shrimp turn pink, about ten minutes.

6. Serve the mixture over your chosen noodles. Only use half of a cup of butternut squash noodles or one cup of spaghetti squash.

Burrito Bowls

This recipe makes four servings. One standard serving has 380 calories, 13 g net carbs, 24 g fat, and 22 g protein.

What you need:

Shredded cheddar cheese, .5 c

Sour cream, .5 c

Guacamole, 1.5 c

Cilantro, .33 c

Diced tomatoes, 2

Lettuce, 340 grams

Salt, 2 tsp.

Olive oil, 2 tbsp.

Cauliflower rice, 3 c

Water, 1 c

Chili powder, 1 tsp.

Cumin, .5 tsp.

Minced garlic, 3 cloves

Diced onion, 1

Paprika, .5 tsp.

Sea salt, 3 tsp.

Juice and zest of a lime

Beef tips, .5 lb.

What you do:

1. In a pressure cooker, add the beef tips, water, paprika, cumin, chili powder, garlic, onion, salt, and lime. Place the pressure cooker on high pressure and let it cook for 20 minutes. Allow all of the pressure to release naturally, or wait ten minutes before using the manual pressure release.

2. Cauliflower rice can be found in the frozen food aisle and the produce department. You can also rice your own if you want. Place the cauliflower

on a parchment lined baking sheet, toss with some oil and two teaspoons of salt, and pat it down so that it is flat. Roast for 15 minutes at 400. Stir, and then cook for another five minutes.

3. To serve everything, place the rice and the meat in a bowl and then top everything with the cold ingredients.

Salami Basil Pizza

This recipe makes four servings. One standard serving has 409 calories, 8 g net carbs, 30 g fat, and 27 g protein.

What you need:

Olive oil, 1 tbsp.

Pepper, .25 tsp.

Salt, .5 tsp.

Sliced basil, 10 leaves

Chopped Hormel Natural Choice salami, 4 sliced

Shredded mozzarella, 3 c

Victoria's marinara sauce, .5 c

Italian seasoning, 1 tsp.

Egg, 1

Parmesan or mozzarella cheese, .5 c

Cauliflower rice, 6 c

What you do:

1. Place your oven to 400. Line a baking sheet with parchment paper.

2. Pour the cauliflower rice on the baking sheet and allow it to cook for 15 minutes.

3. Once the cauliflower has cooled for about five minutes, place it on some cheesecloth. Form it into a ball in the middle of the cloth and squeeze out the liquid. Try to squeeze out as much liquid as you can. The crust will hold up better the dryer you can make the cauliflower.

4. Turn the oven up to 450.

5. Mix together the cauliflower, mozzarella or parmesan, seasonings, and egg.

6. Line a baking sheet with parchment paper. Form four round mini pizza crusts on the pan. Brush the tops of the cuts with olive oil.

7. Allow it to bake for 15 minutes. With a spatula, carefully flip them over and let them cook for five more minutes.

8. At this point, you can allow them to cool completely and store them in a plastic bag in the fridge for up to five days, or you can freeze them for a month.

9. Once you are ready to make your pizzas, allow the crusts to unthaw completely. Top them with the sauce, cheese, salami, and basil. Bake them at 400 until the cheese is golden and bubbly.

Buttercream Fat Bombs

This recipe makes around a dozen fat bombs if you use a traditional cookie scoop, which is about four teaspoons. One standard fat bomb has 138 calories, 5 g net carbs, 14 g fat, and 2 g protein.

What you need:

Lily's dark chocolate, 8 oz.

Vanilla extract, 1 tsp.

Fine salt, .25 tsp.

Sugar-free Truvia, .33 c

Full-fat cream cheese, room temp, .5 c

Grass-fed butter, room temp, .5 c

What you do:

1. Mix together the vanilla, salt, sweetener, cream cheese, and butter until fully combined. You want to make sure that everything is well mixed; otherwise, you could end up with clumps of salt and vanilla.

2. Chill for at least two hours, and then scoop out with a small cookie scoop. Place on a pan and allow to chill for another hour.

3. Melt the chocolate, and then dip the fat bombs into it. Chill until set, about two hours.

Pistachio Almond Fat Bombs

This recipe makes 20 servings. One serving has 202 calories, 1.8 g net carbs, 21 g fat, and 1.7 g protein.

What you need:

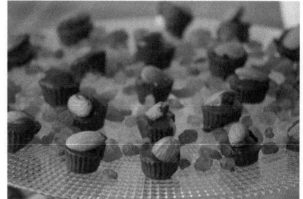

Coconut butter, .5 c

Almond butter, .5 c

Chopped pistachios, 3 tbsp.

Ground cinnamon, .5 tsp.

Salt, .25 tsp.

Ground nutmeg, .25 tsp.

Ground cardamom, .25 tsp.

Pepper, .25 tsp.

Vanilla, 1 tsp.

Sugar-free Truvia, .25 c

Softened butter, 2 tbsp.

Chilled full-fat coconut milk, .25 c

Melted cacao butter, .25 c

Firm coconut oil, .25 c

What you do:

1. Line a 9-inch square dish with parchment paper.

2. Place all of the ingredients in a blender, except for the pistachios and cacao butter. Blend everything together on high until the ingredients are fully combined and airy.

3. Pour the cacao butter in and continue to blend until well incorporated.

4. Pour into the pan and sprinkle the top with the pistachios. Chill overnight.

5. Slice into 20 squares.

Bacon Deviled Eggs

This makes 12 deviled eggs. Two deviled egg has 193 calories, 0 g net carbs, 17 g fat, and 8 g protein.

What you need:

Mayonnaise, .25 c

Cooked bacon, 3 slices

Eggs, 6

Salt

Sliced green onions, 1 stalk

Garlic and onion powder, to taste

Dijon mustard, 1 tsp.

What you do:

1. Place the eggs in water and bring to a boil. Allow them to boil for 15 minutes, and then place them in cold water. Allow them to cool completely, and then peel the eggs.

2. Slice them in half and remove the yolks to a bowl. Smash the yolks with a fork until they are fine.

3. Stir in the seasonings, Dijon, and mayonnaise.

4. Scoop the mixture into the egg whites and top with the bacon and green onions.

Week Two

While having a lot of meal choices is nice, every additional recipe you have to cook is going to take up more of your time. In week two, you will find even more recipes, but if you want to limit your prep and planning, you can limit the recipes to around two per meal type. However, it is nice to have more meal options when you start a keto diet because they will likely help to stave off your cravings.

Breakfast:
Bulletproof Coffee

Breakfast Cheese Tacos

Chocolate Shake

Lunch:
Turnip Green Wraps

Bacon Cheeseburger

Cobb Salad

Dinner:
Lemon Butter Chicken with Mac and Cheese

Egg Roll Bowls

Jalapeno Popper Casserole

Snacks:
Red Hot Cauliflower Bites

Raspberry Almond Bark

Lemon Cheesecake Fat Bombs

Chocolate Chip Cookie Dough Fat Bombs

Chocolate Shake

This is great for those who find themselves not as hungry in the morning. It makes one serving that contains 256 calories, 8 g net carbs, 18 g fat, and 10 g protein.

What you need:

Chocolate exogenous ketones, 1 scoop

Cocoa powder, 2 tbsp.

Unsweetened full-fat yogurt, 3 tbsp.

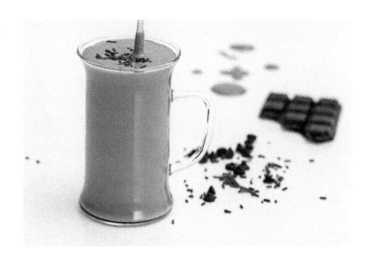

Tahini paste, .5 tbsp.

Stevia drops, 10

Water, .75 c

Egg yolks, 2

What you do:

1. Place all of the ingredients in a blender and pulse until everything is blended.

Cheesy Breakfast Tacos

This makes one serving as has 253 calories, 57 g fat, and 33 g protein.

What you need:

Shredded cheddar cheese, 3 oz.

Egg, 1

Cilantro, 2 sprigs

Salt

Diced tomato, 2 tbsp.

Arugula, .25 c

Grass-fed butter, 1 tsp.

Bacon, 2 slices

What you do:

1. On the day that you prep your meals, back your bacon in the oven at 400 for about 15 minutes. Measure out all of the ingredients that you need so that it is easier to assemble on the day you make this.

2. On the day you want to have the tacos, warm the bacon in the microwave as you prep everything else.

3. Warm a skillet and add the butter. Melt, and then sprinkle in the cheese to make a round taco shell. Once the cheese has melted as is bubbling, crack an egg on top and sprinkle with salt.

4. Once the egg turn opaque and cheese has started to brown, cover with a lid and turn down to low. Allow to cook for another two minutes.

5. Carefully take the taco out of the pan and place it on a cutting board. With two bowls or cups, use them to form the cheese into the shape of a shell. Let it cool until hard.

6. Add in the cilantro, tomato, arugula, and bacon.

Bulletproof Coffee

One standard serving has 474 calories, 3 g net carbs, 45.6 g fat, and 15 g protein.

What you need:

Pumpkin pie spice, .5 tsp. (optional)

Sugar-free Swerve, 1 tsp.

Collagen, 1 tbsp.

Full-fat coconut milk, 2 tbsp.

Ghee, 1 tbsp.

3 egg yolks

MCT oil, 1 tbsp.

Hot coffee, 8 oz.

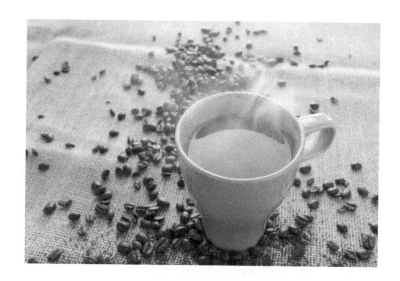

What you do:

1. Place everything in a blender and mix until frothy and smooth.

Cobb Salad

You can't completely make this in advance; you can still prep the majority of the ingredients to save time later in the week. This recipe is one serving and has 901 calories, 8 g net carbs, 50 g fat, and 50 g protein.

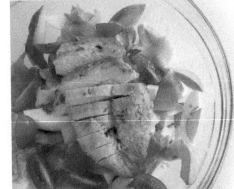

What you need:

Tessemae's Lemon Garlic salad dressing, 2 tbsp.

Shredded cheddar cheese, .25 c

Sliced hardboiled egg

Sliced avocado, .5

Chopped cooked bacon, 1 slice

Sliced cooked chicken thigh

Chopped and washed romaine lettuce, 4 c

What you do:

1. Place all of the ingredients in a bowl and toss with the salad dressing.

Bacon Cheeseburger

This recipe makes one burger and has 485 calories, 9 g net carbs, 65 g fat, and 50 g protein.

What you need:

Iceberg lettuce, several large leaves

Sliced tomato, .5

Mayonnaise, 1 tbsp.

Cheddar cheese, 1 slice

Bacon, 2 slices

Salt, .5 tsp.

Pepper

Garlic powder, .25 tsp.

Onion powder, .25 tsp.

Ground beef, .33 lb.

What you do:

1. Cook the bacon to your desired doneness. Set aside, but make sure you keep the bacon grease. Mix together the pepper, salt, onion powder, garlic powder, and ground beef as the bacon cooks. Form the beef into a patty.

2. Turn up the heat on the pan with the bacon grease. You can grill the burger if you would like. Cook for four minutes on each side. When you are cooking the second side, you can place the cheese slice on the burger to let it melt.

3. Get the veggies prepped as your burger cooks. Pat the lettuce dry.

4. To assemble the burgers, place one or two lettuce leaves on a plate and spread on the mayonnaise. Add on the burger and then the bacon. Finally, top with a couple more lettuce leaves.

Turnip Green Wraps

This makes one wrap and has 594 calories, 7 g net carbs, 55 g fat, and 34 g protein.

What you need:

Keto mayonnaise, 1 tbsp.

Sliced turkey or chicken, 4 oz.

Sliced avocado, .5

Cooked bacon, 2 slices

Sliced Roma tomato, 1

Large, washed, turnip green leaves, 2

What you do:

1. Remove the excess tough stem from the base of the turnip greens. You want to leave most of the stem on the turnip green.

2. Smear the mayonnaise on the leaves and layer on the meat, bacon, avocado, and tomato.

3. Wrap up and enjoy.

Jalapeno Popper Casserole

This whole thing can easily be made ahead of time and store either in the freezer or the fridge until you want to enjoy it. This makes three servings, and each serving has 482 calories, 3 g net carbs, 38 g fat, and 26 g protein

What you need:

Pepper, .25 tsp.

Onion powder, .75 tsp.

Sea salt, .5 tsp. + .5 tsp.

Minced garlic, 2 cloves

Monterey jack cheese, .25 c

Cheddar cheese, .25 c

Heavy cream, 2 tbsp.

Full-fat cream cheese, 3 oz.

Cooked and crumbled bacon, 3 slices

Jalapeno peppers, 3

Boneless and skinless chicken thighs, 12 oz.

What you do:

1. Start by setting your oven to 400 and grease a 9-inch square pan.

2. Chop the chicken thighs into one-inch cubes. Heat up an oiled pan and add in the chicken. Season with pepper and half of the salt.

3. As the chicken is cooking, prep the jalapenos by removing their seeds. Mince two of the jalapenos up and slice the third into rounds.

4. Once the chicken has cooked completely, stir in the cream cheese and heavy cream. Mix until well combined.

5. Stir in the minced jalapeno, three quarters of the crumbled bacon, the Monterey jack cheese, and half of the cheddar. Stir until the cheese has melted and is combined with the other ingredients. Add in the rest of the salt, onion, and garlic. Stir until combined and set it off the heat.

6. Pour the mixture into the prepared pan. Top everything with the remaining cheddar, sliced jalapenos, and bacon.

7. Bake the dish for ten minutes and then flip the oven up to broiler. Allow it to cook for two more minutes until the cheese begins to turn golden and bubble.

Egg Roll Bowls

This recipe makes four servings, and each has 453 calories, 7 g net carbs, 30 g fat, and 33 g protein.

What you need:

Sesame seeds, 2 tbsp.

Salt, 2 tsp.

Coconut aminos, 3 tbsp.

Rice vinegar, 1 tbsp.

Ground ginger, 5 tsp.

Coleslaw mix, 14 oz.

Red chili flakes, 1 tsp.

Ground beef, .5 lb.

Ground pork, .5 lb.

Sliced green onions, 4 stalks

Minced garlic, 4 cloves

Diced onion, 1 med

Sesame oil, 2 tbsp.

What you do:

1. Heat up a pan and add in the sesame oil, white portion of the green onions, garlic, and onion. Sauté everything until the garlic is fragrant and the onions have turned translucent.

2. Add in the salt, ginger, red pepper flakes, beef, and pork. Cook everything until the meat is fully cooked.

3. Stir in the rice vinegar, coconut aminos, and coleslaw mix. Allow it to cook until the coleslaw has become tender.

4. Serve topped with the green part of the green onions and sesame seeds.

Lemon Butter Chicken

This can be fully fixed ahead of time and stored in the fridge for a week or the freezer for a month. This makes two servings, and a single serving has 713 calories, 6 g net carbs, 55 g fat, and 47 g protein.

What you need:

Sea salt, 1 tsp.

Baby spinach, 1 c

Thyme, .25 tsp.

Minced garlic, 3 cloves

Lemon juice, 2 tbsp.

Lemon zest, 1 tsp.

Paprika, 1 tsp.

Grass-fed butter, 2 tbsp.

Parmesan cheese, 2 tbsp.

Chicken broth, 5 c

Heavy cream, .25 c

Bone-in with skin chicken thighs, 2

What you do:

1. Start by placing your oven to 400.

2. Rub your chicken with paprika and sea salt. Heat a cast iron skillet and add in a tablespoon of butter. Place the chicken in the pan sear for three minutes on both sides.

3. Remove the chicken and set aside.

4. Add the rest of the butter and garlic. Cook until fragrant.

5. Stir in the lemon zest, juice, thyme, and chicken broth. Bring up to a boil and allow it to thicken for about seven minutes.

6. Turn the heat down and stir in the heavy cream and parmesan. Allow it to cook for a few more minutes.

7. Mix in the spinach, and cook until the sauce thickens and the spinach has wilted. Place the chicken back in the pan.

8. Place the chicken in the oven and let it cook for 25 minutes, or until it reaches 165.

Mac and Cheese

This makes four servings, and each contains 283 calories, 6 g net carbs, 23 g fat, and 11 g protein.

What you need:

Salt, 2 tsp.

Pepper, .25 tsp.

Turmeric, .5 tsp.

Garlic powder, .5 tsp.

Onion powder, .5 tsp.

Dijon mustard, .5 tsp.

Heavy cream, .5 c

Full-fat cream cheese, cubed, 4 oz.

Sharp shredded cheddar cheese, 4 oz.

Microwave steam bag cauliflower florets, 1 lb.

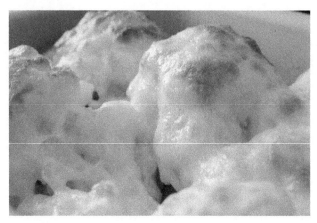

What you do:

1. Cook the cauliflower according to the directions on the package.

2. Add the heavy cream to a pan and let it come to a simmer. Add in the cream cheese and stir until it is melted. Add in two-thirds of the cheddar and mix until melted.

3. Add in all of the seasonings and mix completely. Stir in the cauliflower until coated.

4. Sprinkle with the rest of the cheese and stir until combined.

Chocolate Chip Cookie Dough Fat Bombs

This makes 39 fat bombs, and each fat bomb contains 56 calories, .5 g net carbs, 5.5 g fat, and 1 g protein.

What you need:

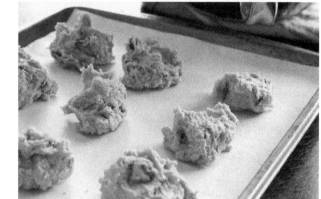

Salt, .25 tsp.

Vanilla, 1 tsp.

Lily's dark chocolate chips, .25 c

Almond butter, .5 c

Sugar-free Truvia, 3 tbsp.

Perfect keto powdered MCT oil, 6 scoops

Full-fat softened cream cheese, 6 tbsp.

Grass-fed butter, 6 tbsp.

What you do:

1. Blend together the butter and cream cheese in a blender. Mix in the salt, vanilla, almond butter, sweetener, and MCT powder until completely combined.

2. Fold in the chocolate chips.

3. Freeze for 10 to 15 minutes.

4. Scoop the mixture out on wax paper with a small cookie scoop.

5. Place back in the freezer until set and place them in a container and keep in the freezer.

Lemon Cheesecake Fat Bombs

This makes 12 servings, and each contains 101 calories, .3 g net carbs, 11 g fat, and .6 g protein.

What you need:

Salt

Sugar-free Truvia, 2-4 tbsp.

Lemon zest, 1 tbsp.

Lemon juice, 2 tsp.

Melted coconut oil, .25 c

Softened grass-fed butter, .25 c

Softened full-fat cream cheese, 4 oz.

What you do:

1. Combine the butter and cream cheese with an electric mixer until airy and smooth.

2. Add in the oil, lemon juice, lemon zest, salt, and sweetener. Combine everything together well with a hand mixer.

3. Pour into 12 silicone molds or a glass pan.

4. Freeze for four to eight hours. Top with extra zest if you want. If you use a glass pan, cut them into 12 squares.

5. These should be kept in the fridge or the freezer.

Raspberry Almond Bark

This will make 16 servings, and one serving contains 186 calories, 4.5 g net carbs, 15 g fat, and 4.4 g protein.

What you need:

Salt, .25 tsp.

Stevia, .5 tsp.

Cocoa powder, 2 tbsp.

Frozen raspberries, .5 c

Chopped and toasted walnuts, 40 grams

Chopped and toasted almonds, 40 grams

Softened coconut butter, 1 c

Almond butter, 1 c

What you do:

1. Place parchment into a 9 x 13 pan.

2. Using a blender, mix together the almond and coconut butter. Once it is combined, add in the cocoa powder, salt, and stevia.

3. In the pan, add the chocolate mixture, and then top it with nuts.

4. Place the frozen raspberries in the microwave for a minute so that they become mushy. Scatter over the top of the chocolate along with the almonds and walnuts.

5. Place the bark in the freezer for no less than an hour. Break into 16 equal size pieces of bark and keep stored in the freezer.

Red Hot Cauliflower Bites

This makes two servings, and each serving contains 222 calories, 5 g net carbs, 21 g fat, and 4 g protein.

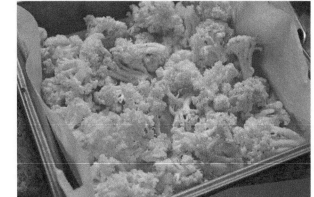

What you need:

Blue cheese dressing, 4 tbsp.

Sea salt, 1 tsp.

Melted grass-fed butter, 1 tbsp.

Garlic powder, 1 tsp.

Hot sauce, .33 c

Cauliflower florets, 1 head or 3 c

What you do:

1. Set your oven to 400. Place parchment on a baking sheet.

2. Mix together the sea salt, garlic powder, hot sauce, and melted butter. Add in the cauliflower and toss it all together.

3. Place on the baking sheet and roast for 18 to 20 minutes.

4. Serve with blue cheese or ranch dressing.

Week Three

Congratulations on making it through the first two weeks. By now, you have probably figured out which dishes you like the best and which ones you will incorporate into your regular diet. You will also probably know how many different meals you are comfortable with meal prepping for the week.

This is your third and final week. After this, you can come up with your own menu by combining the recipes from these three weeks and the other recipes that you will find in the rest of the book. You will find what works best for you.

Breakfast:

Cream Cheese Danish

Hash Browns, Bacon, and Eggs

Chai Tea Latte

Lunch:

Broccoli Cheddar Soup

Chicken Salad

Lasagna Bowls

Dinner:

Beef Stroganoff Meatballs with Noodles

Butter Salmon with Capers and Zucchini Gratin

Chicken Cordon Bleu Casserole

Snacks:

Peppermint Mocha Drops

Mocha Bonbons

Broccoli Cheddar Tots

Chai Tea Latte

You can prepare a large batch of the spice mixture to make things faster when you fix this. One standard serving has 254 calories, 8 g net carbs, 68 g fat, and 5 g protein.

What you need:

Latte

Chair blend, 1 tsp.

Black tea, 2 bags

Sugar-free Truvia, 2 tsp.

Grass-fed butter, 1 tbsp.

Full-fat coconut milk, 8 oz.

Chair Blend

Ground nutmeg, 1 tsp.

Pepper, .25 tsp.

Ground cinnamon, 1 tbsp.

Ground cardamom, 2 tsp.

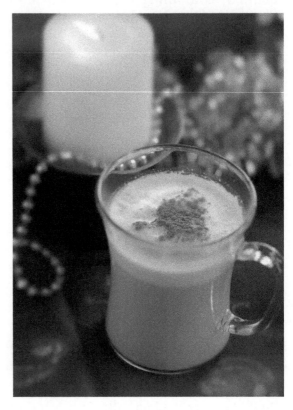

What you do:

1. Heat the coconut milk and butter in the microwave for two minutes.

2. Once hot, add in the tea bags and let it brew for four minutes.

3. Discard the tea and add to the blender along with the chai blend and sweetener. Blend for a few seconds until frothy.

Hash Browns, Bacon, and Eggs

It makes three servings of hash browns but one serving of eggs and bacon. A single serving of this has 516 calories, 10 g net carbs, 40 g fat, and 27 g protein.

What you need:

Hash browns, 2

Slice of bacon

Cooked egg

Hash brown

Melted butter, 1 tbsp.

Pepper

Sea salt, .5 tsp.

Garlic powder, .25 tsp.

Onion powder, .25 tsp.

Egg

Shredded cheese, .75 c

Cauliflower rice, 3 c

What you do:

1. Add the cauliflower to a bowl and cover with a damp paper towel. Microwave for 2.5 minutes. Allow it to cool slightly.

2. Once cooled, place in a cheesecloth and squeeze out as much liquid as you can.

3. Place back into the bowl and add in the seasonings, egg, and cheese. Mix everything together.

4. Portion the mixture into six rectangles on a baking sheet. Brush them with melted butter.

5. Bake for 15 minutes, flip them and then bake for another five. Take them out of the oven and sprinkle with some salt.

6. Keep stored in the freezer.

7. Heat two up with your bacon and egg for a delicious breakfast.

Cream Cheese Danish

These can be made in advance and stored in the fridge for a week. Microwave for a few seconds to heat up. This makes four danishes, and each contains 523 calories, 9 g net carbs, 40 g fat, and 19 g protein.

What you need:

Baking powder, .5 tsp.

Sea salt, .25 tsp.

Vanilla, .5 tsp.

Egg

Melted butter, 4 tbsp.

Sugar-free Truvia, 2 tbsp.

Almond flour, 6 tbsp.

Coconut flour, 3 tbsp.

Block of mozzarella, 140 grams

Filling

Thawed frozen raspberries or blackberries, .25 c

Sugar-free Truvia, 5 tbsp.

Egg yolk

Vanilla, .5 tsp.

Lemon juice, 1 tsp.

Softened full-fat cream cheese, 6 oz.

What you do:

1. Mix all of the filling ingredients together, minus the berries. Mix with a hand mixer until light and fluffy. Set in the fridge until ready for use.

2. Set your oven to 400. Line a baking sheet with parchment.

3. Mix together the coconut flour, almond flour, baking powder, and salt. Mix in the butter, vanilla, and sweetener. Stir until combined.

4. Shred the mozzarella. Melt in the microwave for a couple of minutes.

5. Mix the cheese into the flour mixture. Once everything is combined, stir in the egg yolk.

6. Microwave for 10 seconds and then knead together until combined and is of an even color.

7. Roll the dough on the parchment paper and separate into four squares.

8. Spoon the filling into the middle of the squares and top with the berries.

9. Fold the four corners of the square into the center.

10. Bake for 10 to 13 minutes. Pull them out once they are golden in color. They will burn easily.

Chicken Salad

This makes two servings, and each has 406 calories, 4 g net carbs, 28 g fat, and 31 g protein.

What you need:

Salt, .5 tsp.

Butterhead lettuce, 1 head

Garlic powder, .25 tsp.

Onion powder, .25 tsp.

Sour cream, .25 c

Mayonnaise, 2 tbsp.

Thinly sliced celery, 1 stalk

Shredded cheddar cheese, .25 c

Chopped, cooked bacon, 2 slices

Cubed or shredded chicken, 1 c

What you do:

1. Mix all of the ingredients, except for the lettuce, together. Serve the chicken mixture over the lettuce.

Lasagna Bowls

This is a single serving recipe and contains 620 calories, 7 g net carbs, 51 g fat, and 30 g protein.

What you need:

Italian seasoning, .25 tsp.

Pepper

Salt, .25 tsp.

Parmesan cheese, 2 tbsp.

Mozzarella, 2 tbsp.

Full-fat ricotta cheese, .25 c

Marinara sauce, .25 c

Cooked Italian sausage, 4 oz.

What you do:

1. Add the sausage to a microwave-safe bowl.

2. Drop in the ricotta and sprinkle on the seasonings. Pour in the marinara sauce and top with the remaining cheeses.

3. Microwave for two minutes until hot and bubbly.

Broccoli Cheddar Soup

This makes two servings, and each contains 53 calories, 4 g net carbs, 46 g fat, and 25 g protein.

What you need:

Chopped broccoli florets, 1.5 c

Olive oil, 1 tbsp.

Minced garlic, 2 cloves

Sea salt, 1 tsp.

 Pepper, .25 tsp.

Chicken brother, 1.75 c

Heavy cream, .5 c

Shredded cheddar cheese, 1.5 c

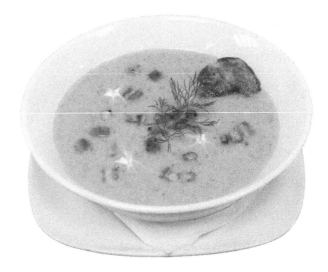

What you do:

1. Add the olive oil and garlic to a pot and sauté until fragrant.

2. Add in the broccoli florets, broth, and cream. Bring to a boil, reduce heat, and simmer until tender. The time this takes will vary on how small the broccoli is, but it should be around 10 to 20 minutes.

3. Slowly stir in the shredded cheese. Make sure you stir constantly. Don't add the cheese all at once. Slowly add it in so that it melts correctly.

4. Once the cheese has melted, remove from heat. This can be stored in the fridge or freezer.

Chicken Cordon Bleu Casserole

This can be made in advance and stored in the fridge or freezer until needed. It makes four servings, and each contains: 574 calories, 3 g net carbs, 34 g fat, and 59 g protein.

What you need:

Minced garlic, 2 cloves

Dijon mustard, 2 tsp.

Sliced Swiss cheese, 3 oz.

Melted butter, .25 c + 1 tbsp.

Softened full-fat cream cheese, 3 oz.

Sliced ham, 3 oz.

Sliced or cubed chicken, 1 lb.

Sea salt, 1 tsp.

Lemon juice, 3 tbsp.

Diced onion, .25 c

What you do:

1. Set your oven to 350 and grease a 9-inch baking dish.

2. Add the onion and butter to a pan. Cook until they are translucent, about five minutes. Stir in the garlic and cook until fragrant.

3. In a blender, mix together the salt, lemon juice, Dijon, cream cheese, and butter until smooth.

4. Add the chicken to the baking dish, add in the onion mixture, and then the ham. Spread over the sauce.

5. Lay the Swiss cheese on top and let it bake for 35 minutes.

6. Turn up to the broiler and bake for two minutes until bubbly and golden. Allow it to sit for a few minutes before serving.

Butter Salmon

This makes two servings, and one serving has 532 calories, 1 g net carbs, 29 g fat, and 65 g protein.

What you need:

Salt, 1 tsp.

Pepper, .25 tsp.

Capers, 1 tbsp.

Minced garlic, 2 cloves

Lemon zest, .5 tsp.

Lemon juice, 1 tbsp.

Butter, 3 tbsp.

Salmon fillets, 2

Paprika, .25 tsp.

What you do:

1. Set your oven to 400.

2. Add the butter and garlic to a large skillet. Cook until it becomes fragrant. Add in the lemon zest and juice.

3. Add the salmon to the pan and sprinkle with paprika, pepper, and salt.

4. Bake until the salmon is cooked all the way through, around 15 minutes. Around five minutes before it is done, add in the capers and add bake to the oven. Serve with the cheesy zucchini gratin.

Cheesy Zucchini Gratin

This makes two servings. Each serving has 298 calories, 6 g net carbs, 25 g fat, and 12 g protein.

What you need:

Pepper, .25 tsp.

Sea salt, 1 tsp.

Shredded pepper jack cheese, .75 c

Butter, 1 tbsp.

Heavy cream, .25 c

Minced garlic, 3 cloves

Sliced onion

Zucchini rounds, 2 c

What you do:

1. Set your oven to 375. Grease an 8-inch baking pan.

2. Add a third of the zucchini and the sliced onion into the baking pan and sprinkle with some salt and pepper. Top with a quarter cup of shredded cheese.

3. Repeat these layers two more times until you have used all of the onion and zucchini.

4. Melt the butter and stir in the garlic until fragrant. Pour this into the heavy cream. Allow to simmer.

5. Pour this over the veggies. Place in the oven and bake until it has turned golden and thickened, about 35 to 40 minutes.

Beef Stroganoff Meatballs with Noodles

This makes three servings, and each serving contains 492 calories, 14 g net carbs, 39 g fat, and 19 g protein.

What you need:

Garlic powder, .5 tsp.

Pepper, .25 tsp.

Almond flour, 3 tbsp.

Egg

Ground beef, .5 lb.

Sea salt, 1 tsp.

Worcestershire sauce, 1 tsp.

Dried parsley, .5 tsp.

Onion powder, .5 tsp.

Sauce

Konjac noodles, 2 servings

Xanthan gum, pinch

Pepper, .25 tsp.

Sea salt, 1 tsp.

Sour cream, .33 c

Beef broth, .75 c

Minced garlic, 3 cloves

Sliced onion, 1 med

Sliced mushrooms, 8 oz.

Butter, 2 tbsp.

What you do:

1. Set your oven to 400. Place parchment on a baking sheet.

2. Mix all of the meatball ingredients together and use an ice cream scoop to shape it into balls. Place them on the baking sheet. Bake for 10 minutes.

3. Meanwhile, add the butter to a pan. Add in the onions and cook until translucent. Add in the mushrooms and cook for seven minutes. Mix in the garlic until fragrant.

4. Add the broth, xanthan gum, pepper, salt, and sour cream. Allow this mixture to come to a simmer.

5. Add in the cooked meatballs. Place a lid on the pan and allow it to simmer for 20 minutes.

6. Serve this over top of konjac noodles.

Broccoli Cheddar Tots

This makes two servings, and each contains 319 calories, 7 g net carbs, 22 g fat, and 21 g protein.

What you need:

Cooking spray

Sea salt, 1 tsp.

Almond flour, .25 c

Coconut flour, 2 tbsp.

Diced onion, .25 c

Parmesan, .25 c

Sharp cheddar cheese, .5 c

Eggs, 2

Broccoli florets, 2 c

What you do:

1. Set your oven to 400 and line a baking sheet with parchment paper.

2. Place the broccoli in a microwave-safe and cover with a damp towel. Microwave two minutes.

3. Chop up the broccoli and then add back to the bowl. Add in the rest of the ingredients and combine completely.

4. With a tablespoon scoop, portion out the broccoli into tot forms.

5. Place the tots on a baking sheet and spray them with cooking spray and bake for six minutes. Flip, and bake for seven minutes.

Mocha Bonbons

This will make 15 bonbons, and each of the bonbons contains 112 calories, 2.6 g net carbs, 13.4 g fat, and 6 g protein.

What you need:

Coffee beans, 15 pieces

Cocoa butter, 2 tbsp.

MCT oil, 3 tbsp.

Dark chocolate chips, .66 c

Cocoa, 2 tbsp.

Sugar-free Truvia, .25 c

Strong coffee, .25 c

Softened full-fat cream cheese, 8 oz.

What you do:

1. Add the cream cheese to a bowl along with the cocoa, sweetener, and coffee. Blend with an electric mixer until fluffy and combined. Chill for four hours or overnight.

2. With a small cookie scoop, scoop the mixture into balls on wax paper. Let them freeze for half an hour.

3. Melt the chocolate with the cocoa butter and MCT oil in the microwave. Cover the truffles with the chocolate and top with a single coffee bean. Freeze for an hour, and store in an airtight container.

Peppermint Mocha Drops

This will make six drops, and each contains 183 calories, 3 g net carbs, 19 g fat, and 0 g protein.

What you need:

Vanilla, .5 tsp.

Peppermint extract, 2 tsp.

Liquid stevia, 40 drops

Melted dark chocolate baking chips, .33 c

Softened butter, .25 c

Softened coconut oil, .25 c

What you do:

1. Place all of the ingredients in a blender and combine until smooth and homogenous.

2. Scoop the mixture into small silicone baking cups. It should be about two tablespoons of the mixture.

3. Freeze until hard, about 15 minutes, and keep stored in the fridge or the freezer.

4. When you want, blend into a cup of hot coffee.

Chapter 10: Breakfast

Peanut Butter Cup Smoothie

This makes two servings and per serving contains 486 calories, 6 g net carbs, 30 g protein, and 40 g fat.

What you need:

- Peanut butter, 2 tbsp.

- Chocolate protein powder, 1 scoop

- Coconut cream, .75 c

- Water, 1 c

- Ice cubes, 3

What you do:

1. Place all of the ingredients in a strong blender and mix everything together until smooth.

2. Pour the mixture into two glasses.

Breakfast Bake

This makes eight servings, and each serving contains 303 calories, 3 g net carbs, 24 g fat, and 17 g protein.

What you need:

- Shredded cheddar cheese, .5 c

- Pepper

- Salt

- Chopped oregano, 1 tbsp.

- Cooked spaghetti squash, 2 c

- Eggs, 8

- Sausage, 1 lb.

- Olive oil, 1 tbsp.

What you do:

1. Set your oven to 375 and grease a 9 x 13 casserole dish.

2. Add the olive oil to a large ovenproof skillet and heat up.

3. Add the sausage and cook thoroughly around five minutes. As the sausage is cooking, beat the eggs together along with the oregano and squash. Season it with some pepper and salt.

4. Mix the sausage into the egg mixture. Stir everything together until combined and pour into your prepared casserole dish.

5. Sprinkle the top with the cheese and cover it loosely with foil.

6. Slide the casserole into the oven for 30 minutes, and then take the foil off and let it cook for another 15 minutes.

7. Allow to sit for ten minutes before you serve it.

Mushroom Frittata

This makes six servings, and each serving contains 316 calories, 1 g net carbs, 27 g fat, and 16 g protein.

What you need:

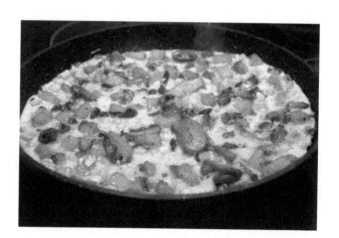

- Pepper

- Salt

- Crumbled goat cheese, .5 c

- Beaten eggs, 10

- Chopped and cooked bacon, 6 slices

- Shredded spinach, 1 c

- Sliced mushrooms, 1 c

- Olive oil, 2 tbsp.

What you do:

1. Start by placing your oven to 350.

2. Heat the olive oil in a large ovenproof pan.

3. Sauté the mushrooms until they are browned lightly, around three minutes.

4. Add the bacon and spinach to the pan and sauté until the greens have wilted.

5. Add the beaten eggs. Don't stir. Allow the eggs to set, and life the edges up every so often to let the uncooked egg to flow underneath. Cook for around three to four minutes.

6. Sprinkle goat cheese on top and season with some pepper and salt.

7. Bake the frittata until it has fully set and browned, about 15 minutes.

8. Remove and allow to sit for five minutes. Slice into six wedges and serve.

Avocado and Eggs

This makes four servings, and each serving contains 324 calories, 3 g net carbs, 25 g fat, 19 g protein.

What you need:

- Pepper

- Salt

- Cheddar cheese, .25 c

- Cooked and shredded chicken breast, 4 oz.

- Eggs, 4

- Avocados, 2

What you do:

1. Start by placing the oven to 425.

2. Slice the avocados in half and remove the pits. Scoop out a bit of the flesh from the avocado so that it is about twice as big as it was.

3. Lay the halves into an 8-inch square baking dish with the fleshy side up.

4. Crack on egg into each of the holes in the avocado halves. Divide the shredded chicken between the halves and sprinkle the tops of them with cheese. Season them with a little bit of pepper and salt.

5. Slide them into the oven and cook until the eggs are cooked to your desired doneness, about 15 to 20 minutes.

Creamy Cinnamon Smoothie

This makes two servings, and each serving contains 492 calories, 6 g net carbs, 47 g fat, and 18 g protein.

What you need:

- Vanilla, .5 tsp.

- Ground cinnamon, 1 tsp.

- Liquid stevia, 5 drops

- Vanilla protein powder, 1 scoop

- Coconut milk, 2 c

What you do:

1. Add all of the ingredients to your blender and mix until everything is smooth and incorporated.

2. Divide the mixture between two glasses.

Everything Bagel

This makes 12 servings, and each serving contains 25 calories, .5 g net carbs, 2 g fat, 3 g protein.

What you need:

- Everything bagel seasoning

- Smoked salmon, 4 oz.

- Full-fat butter, 1 tbsp.

- Full-fat cream cheese, 4 oz.

What you do:

1. Mix together the salmon, butter, and cream cheese together until it is evenly distributed. You don't want to have clumps of each ingredient. You want everything to be smooth.

2. Place in the refrigerator for 30 minutes. Allow the mixture to stiffen up a bit.

3. Once it has become firmer, divide the mixture into 12 equal portions and roll into balls.

4. Finally, roll the balls in some of the everything bagel seasonings. If you don't want to use salmon, you can also use bacon.

5. When you keep them refrigerated, the bagels will keep a firmer consistency and are easy to grab in the morning when you don't have time to cook.

Nut Medley Granola

This makes eight servings, and each serving contains 391 calories, 4 g net carbs, 38 g fat, and 10 g protein.

What you need:

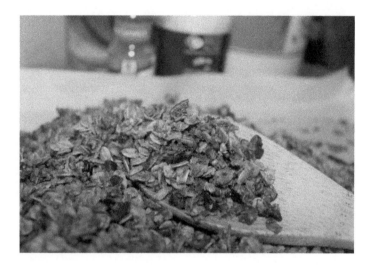

- Ground nutmeg, .5 tsp.

- Ground cinnamon, 1 tsp.

- Liquid Stevia, 10 drops

- Melted coconut oil, .5 c, melted

- Walnuts, .5 c

- Pumpkin seeds, .5 c, raw

- Sunflower seeds, 1 c, raw

- Shredded unsweetened coconut, 2 c

- Sliced almonds, 1 c

What you do:

6. Heat up your oven to 250 degrees. Take two large baking sheets and line them with parchment paper. Set this to the side.

7. Add the walnuts, pumpkin seeds, sunflower seeds, almonds, and shredded coconut to a large bowl and toss until mixed well.

8. Add the nutmeg, cinnamon, stevia, and coconut oil to a small bowl and mix until well blended.

9. Pour this mixture over the nuts and seeds. Using your hands, toss the nuts until they have been well coated with the coconut mixture.

10. Divide the granola between the two baking sheets and spread evenly.

11. Bake for one hour. Stir the granola every 15 minutes until crunchy and golden.

12. Remove from oven and allow to cool. Break up any large chunks into bite-size pieces.

13. Store in an airtight container. This can be stored in the freezer or refrigerator for one month.

Berry Green Smoothie

This makes two servings, and each serving contains 436 calories, 6 g net carbs, 36 g fat, and 28 g protein.

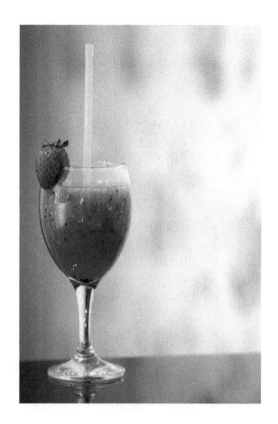

What you need:

- Vanilla protein powder, 1 scoop

- Coconut oil, 1 tbsp.

- Cream cheese, .75 c

- Kale, .5 c, shredded

- Raspberries, .5 tsp.

- Water, 1 c

What you do:

1. Place all ingredients into the blender. Blend until smooth and creamy.

2. Pour into glasses and enjoy.

Bacon Artichoke Omelet

This makes four servings, and each serving contains 435 calories, 3 g net carbs, 39 g fat, and 17 g protein.

What you need:

- Pepper

- Salt

- Artichoke hearts, .5 c, canned, packed in water

- Onion, .25 c, chopped

- Olive oil, 1 tbsp.

- Chopped bacon, 8 slices

- Heavy whipping cream, 2 tbsp.

- Eggs, 6 beaten

What you do:

1. Heat up a large skillet and cook the bacon until it is crispy.

2. Remove bacon and drain. Allow to cool for a few minutes.

3. Put heavy cream, bacon, and eggs into a bowl and whisk until well blended. Set to the side.

4. Remove bacon grease from pan and wipe clean. Add olive oil and onion and cook until tender. This will take about three minutes.

5. Pour the egg mixture into the skillet and swirl it around for one minute.

6. Continue to cook, lifting the edges to allow the uncooked egg to glow under for about two minutes.

7. Put the artichoke hearts on top and flip the omelet. Cook an additional four minutes until the egg is firm. Flip again so that the artichoke hearts are back on top.

8. Take off heat, cut into quarters and season generously with pepper and salt. Place on plates and enjoy.

Chapter 11: Main Dishes

Stuffed Chicken Breasts

This makes four servings, and each serving contains 389 calories, 3 g net carbs, 30 g fat, and 25 g protein.

What you need:

- EVOO, 2 tbsp.

- Skin-on chicken breasts, 4-5 oz. breasts

- Chopped basil, 2 tbsp.

- Chopped roasted red pepper, .25 c

- Chopped kalamata olives, .25 c

- Room temp goat cheese, .5 c

- Chopped sweet onion, .25 c

- Butter, 1 tbsp.

What you do:

1. Start by placing your oven to 400.

2. In a small pan, melt the butter and add in the onion. Let the onion cook until tender, around three minutes.

3. Place the onion in a bowl and add in the basil, red pepper, olives, and cheese. Stir everything together until it is all well blended. Refrigerate the mixture for at least 30 minutes.

4. Slice a horizontal pocket into each of the chicken breasts and stuff each evenly with the filling that you made earlier. Secure them with toothpicks.

5. Heat the olive oil in an ovenproof skillet and add in the chicken. Brown the chicken on both sides, about five minutes on each side.

6. Slide the skillet into the oven and cook until the chicken has cooked through, around 15 minutes. Take out the toothpicks before serving.

Roasted Pork Loin with Mustard Sauce

This makes eight servings, and each serving contains 368 calories, 2 g net carbs, 29 g fat, and 25 g protein.

What you need:

- Grainy mustard, 3 tbsp.

- Heavy cream, 1.5 c

- Olive oil, 3 tbsp.

- Pepper

- Salt

- Boneless pork loin roast, 2 lbs.

What you do:

1. Start by placing your oven to 375.

2. Rub your pork roast with pepper and salt.

3. Add the olive oil to a large skillet. Add in the roast and brown on all sides. This should take about six minutes in total. Place the roast into a baking dish.

4. Bake for about an hour, or until the internal temperature reaches 155.

5. When there are around 15 minutes left on the roasting time, add a small pot on medium heat and add the mustard and cream.

6. Stir the sauce until it comes to a simmer. Turn the heat to low and allow it to simmer for five minutes or until it becomes thick. Take the pot off the heat.

7. Allow the pork to rest for ten minutes. Slice and serve topped with the sauce.

Garlic-Braised Short Rib

This makes four servings, and each serving contains 481 calories, 2 g net carbs, 38 g fat, and 29 g protein.

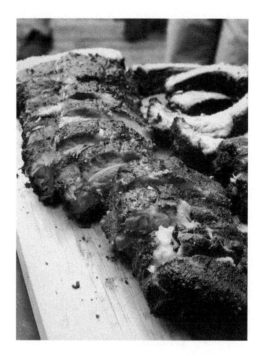

What you need:

- Beef stock, 3 c

- Dry red wine, .5 c

- Minced garlic, 2 tsp.

- Olive oil, 1 tbsp.

- Pepper

- Salt

- Beef short ribs, 4-4 oz. racks

What you do:

1. Start by placing your oven to 325. Rub the ribs with pepper and salt.

2. Grab a deep ovenproof skillet and add in the olive oil and let heat to medium-high.

3. Sear the ribs in the pan on all sides until they are browned. Transfer to a plate.

4. Place the garlic in a skillet and cook until fragrant, around three minutes.

5. Whisk the wine to deglaze your pan. Make sure that you scrap all of the little-browned bits off of the bottom of the pan. Let the wine simmer until it has reduced slightly, about two minutes.

6. Pour in the beef stock, and then add the ribs and any juices they have accumulated. Allow the mixture to come to a boil.

7. Place a lid on the skillet and place it in the oven. Cook the ribs for about two hours. They should be fall-off-the-bone tender.

8. Serve the ribs along with the cooking liquid drizzled over.

Italian Beef Burgers

This makes four servings, and each serving contains 441 calories, 3 g net carbs, 37 g fat, and 22 g protein.

What you need:

- Thinly sliced onion, .25 onion

- Tomato sliced into four slices

- Olive oil, 1 tbsp.

- Salt, .25 tsp.

- Minced garlic, 1 tsp.

- Chopped basil, 2 tbsp.

- Ground almonds, .25 c

- Lean ground beef, 1 lb.

What you do:

1. Combine the salt, garlic, basil, ground almonds, and ground beef together in a bowl.

2. Form the mixture into four equal sized patties and flatten them to about a half-inch thick.

3. Add olive oil to a large skillet and heat to medium-high.

4. Panfry the burger patties until they are cooked through; flip them once during the cooking time. It should take about six minutes on each side.

5. Pay away excess grease and serve along with onion and tomato.

Sirloin with Compound Butter

This makes four servings, and each serving contains 544 calories, 0 g net carbs, 44 g fat, and 35 g protein.

What you need:

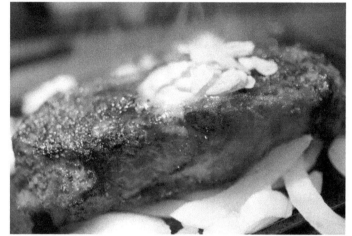

- Pepper

- Salt

- Olive oil, 1 tbsp.

- Beef sirloin steaks, 4-5 oz.

- Blue cheese, 4 oz.

- Room temp butter, 6 tbsp.

What you do:

1. Add the butter to a blender and pulse until it has been whipped up, around two minutes.

2. Add in the cheese, and pulse until well mixed.

3. Spoon out on a sheet of plastic wrap and roll it into a log that is about 1.5 inches in diameter.

4. Refrigerate until it has set up, around an hour.

5. Slice into half inch disks and place on a plate in the refrigerator until you are ready to serve your steaks. Store any of the leftovers in the fridge for up to a week.

6. Heat up your grill. As this is happening, allow the steaks to come up to room temp.

7. Rub the steaks with olive oil, pepper, and salt.

8. Grill the steaks until they are done to your likely. Six minutes on each side will cook it to around medium. If you don't have a grill, you can pan fry or broil the steaks for about seven minutes on each side for medium.

9. Allow the steaks to rest for about ten minutes. Serve each steak along with a disk of butter.

Lamb with Tomato Pesto

This makes eight servings, and each serving contains 352 calories, 3 g net carbs, 29 g fat, and 17 g protein.

What you need:

- Lamb

- Olive oil, 2 tbsp.

- Pepper

- Salt

- Leg of lamb, 2 lb.

- Pesto

- Minced garlic, 2 tsp.

- Chopped basil, 2 tbsp.

- EVOO, 2 tbsp.

- Pine nuts, .25 c

- Sun-dried tomatoes in oil, drained, 1 c

What you do:

1. For the Pesto – Add the garlic, basil, olive oil, pine nuts, and tomatoes to a blender or food processor. Mix up until smooth and then set aside until you need to use it.

2. Leg of Lamb – Start by placing your oven to 400. Rub the lamb with pepper and salt.

3. Add olive oil to an ovenproof pan and heat to medium-high.

4. Sear the lamb on all sides until it is nicely browned.

5. Spread the tomato peas over the lamb and set them on a baking sheet. Slide into the oven and roast until it reaches your desired doneness. An hour of cooking will take it to about medium.

6. Allow the lamb to rest for ten minutes before you serve it.

Lamb Chops with Kalamata Tapenade

This makes four servings, and each serving contains 348 calories, 1 g net carbs, 28 g fat, and 21 g protein.

What you need:

- Lamb Chops

- Olive oil, 1 tbsp.

- Pepper

- Salt

- French-cut lamb chops, 2 1-lb. racks

- Tapenade

- Lemon juice, 2 tsp.

- Minced garlic, 2 tsp.

- EVOO, 2 tbsp.

- Chopped parsley, 2 tbsp.

- Kalamata olives, 1 c

What you do:

1. For the Tapenade – Add the lemon juice, garlic, olive oil, parsley, and olives to a food processor and process until it is pureed but still chunky.

2. Transfer to a container and keep in the fridge until you need it.

3. For the Lamb Chops – Start by placing your oven on 450. Rub the lamb with pepper and salt.

4. Place the oil in an ovenproof skillet and heat up to medium-high. Place the lamb racks on the pan and sear until browned on all sides.

5. Place the racks upright in the skillet. The bones should be interlaced. Roast them in the oven until it has reached your desired doneness. For

medium-rare, cook it for about 20 minutes. The internal temp needs to reach at least 125.

6. Allow the lamb to rest for at least ten minutes. Slice the lamb racks into individual chops. Give four chops per person and top with the tapenade you made earlier.

Herb Butter Scallops

This makes four servings, and each serving contains 306 calories, 4 g net carbs, 24 g fat, and 19 g protein.

What you need:

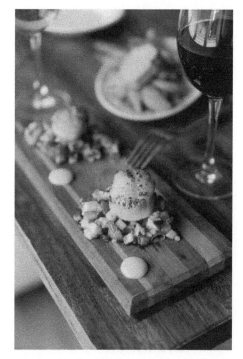

- Chopped basil, 2 tsp.

- Butter, 8 tbsp.

- Pepper

- Chopped thyme, 1 tsp.

- Minced garlic, 2 tsp.

- One lemon juiced

- Cleaned sea scallops, 1 lb.

What you do:

1. Make sure the scallops are completely dry by patting them with paper towels. Season with pepper.

2. Warm a large skillet and add two tablespoons of butter to the skillet.

3. Evenly space the scallops in the skillet. Cook on each side until golden brown. This will take about 2 ½ minutes for each side.

4. Remove from skillet onto a plate and set to the side.

5. Add the rest of the butter to the skillet and add garlic. Sauté for three minutes until garlic is fragrant and translucent.

6. Add in thyme, basil, and lemon juice, stir well. Put the scallops back into the skillet. Flip them over to coat with sauce.

7. Serve and enjoy.

Halibut with Citrus Butter Sauce

This makes four servings, and each serving contains 319 calories, 2 g net carbs, 26 g fat, and 22 g protein.

What you need:

- Olive oil, 2 tbsp.

- Chopped parsley, 2 tsp.

- Orange juice, 1 tbsp.

- Lemon juice, 1 tbsp.

- Dry white wine, 3 tbsp.

- Minced shallot, 1

- Minced garlic, 2 tsp.

- Butter, .25 c

- Pepper

- Halibut fillets, 4-5 oz. fillets

What you do:

1. Make sure the fish is completely dry by patting it with paper towels. Season the fillet with pepper and salt. Place on a plate that has been lined with paper towels.

2. Warm a saucepan and melt the butter.

3. Add in shallot and garlic and cook until tender. This will take three minutes.

4. Add in the orange juice, lemon juice, and white wine and allow the sauce to simmer. Let it cook until it is slightly thickened. This will take about two minutes.

5. Take off heat and add parsley. Set to the side.

6. Warm a large skillet and add olive oil.

7. Fry the fish until lightly browned and cooked through, turning over once. This will take about ten minutes.

8. Place each piece of fish on a plate. Put a spoonful of sauce on each fillet.

Coconut Haddock

This makes four servings, and each serving contains 299 calories, 1 g net carbs, 24 g fat, and 20 g protein.

What you need:

- Melted coconut oil, 2 tbsp.

- Ground hazelnuts, .25 c

- Unsweetened shredded coconut, 1 c

- Pepper

- Salt

- Boneless haddock fillets, 4-5 oz.

What you do:

1. Heat up your oven to 400. Put parchment paper onto a large baking sheet. Set to the side.

2. Make sure the fillets are dry by patting them with paper towels. Season them with pepper and salt.

3. Put the hazelnuts and coconut into a small bowl and stir to mix well.

4. Place the fish fillets into the coconut mixture. Make sure both sides of the fish are coated well.

5. Put the fish on the prepared baking sheet and brush both sides with coconut oil.

6. Bake for 12 minutes or until the topping is golden brown and flakes easily.

7. Serve and enjoy.

Chapter 12: Side Dishes

Asparagus and Walnuts

This makes four servings, and each serving contains 124 calories, 2 g net carbs, 12 g fat, and 3 g protein.

What you need:

- Chopped walnuts, .25 c

- Pepper

- Salt

- Trimmed asparagus, .75 lb.

- Olive oil, 1.5 tbsp.

What you do:

1. Heat a large skillet with some olive oil over medium-high.

2. Add the asparagus and sauté until they are tender and browned lightly. This takes about five minutes.

3. Season with some pepper and salt.

4. Take the pan off the heat and toss the walnuts in with the asparagus.

Creamed Spinach

This makes four servings, and each serving contains 195 calories, 1 g net carbs, 20 g fat, and 3 g protein.

What you need:

- Nutmeg, pinch
- Pepper
- Salt
- Herbed chicken stock, .25 c
- Heavy cream, .75 c
- Stemmed and cleaned spinach, 4 c
- Sliced onion, .5
- Butter, 1 tbsp.

What you do:

1. Add the butter to a large pan. Add in the onion and sauté until lightly browned, around five minutes.
2. Mix in the nutmeg, pepper, salt, chicken stock, heavy cream, and spinach.
3. Cook for about five minutes, or until the spinach has wilted.
4. Continue to cook until the spinach is tender and the sauce has thickened, 15 minutes.

Golden Rosti

This makes eight servings, and each serving contains 171 calories, 3 g net carbs, 15 g fat, and 5 g protein.

What you need:

- Butter, 2 tbsp.

- Pepper

- Salt

- Chopped thyme, 1 tsp.

- Minced garlic, 2 tsp.

- Grated parmesan, 2 tbsp.

- Shredded raw celeriac, 1 c

- Shredded acorn squash, 1 c

- Chopped bacon, 8 slices

What you do:

1. Heat up a large skillet and cook the bacon until it is crispy.

2. As the bacon cooks, combines the thyme, garlic, parmesan, celeriac, and squash. Season it with a generous amount of pepper and salt. Set to the side.

3. Take the bacon out of the pan with a slotted spoon and add to the rosti mixture. Stir everything together.

4. Keep two tablespoons of bacon fat in the skillet and add in the butter.

5. Turn the heat down and add the rosti mixture to the skillet, and spread it out so that it forms a large round patty that is about an inch thick.

6. Cook until the bottom has turned golden and has crisped up.

7. Flip it over and let it cook until the other side is crispy and it is cooked in the middle.

8. Take it out of the pan and slice into eight pieces.

Mushrooms with Camembert

This makes four servings, and each serving contains 161 calories, 3 g net carbs, 13 g fat, and 9 g protein.

What you need:

- Pepper

- Diced camembert cheese, 4 oz.

- Halved button mushrooms, 1 lb.

- Minced garlic, 2 tsp.

- Butter, 2 tbsp.

What you do:

1. Melt the butter in a large skillet on medium-high.

2. Cook the garlic until it becomes fragrant, about three minutes. Add in the mushrooms and cook until tender, about ten minutes. Mix in the cheese. Sauté for two minutes, or until the cheese has melted.

3. Stir in some pepper and enjoy.

Crispy Zucchini

This makes four servings, and each serving contains 94 calories, 1 g net carbs, 8 g fat, and 4 g protein.

What you need:

- Pepper

- Grated parmesan, .5 c

- Zucchini sliced into .25-inch rounds, 4 zucchini

- Butter, 2 tbsp.

What you do:

1. Melt the butter in a large skillet.

2. Add in the zucchini and let it cook until it is tender and browned, around five minutes.

3. Spread the zucchini evenly onto the bottom of the skillet and sprinkle the top of the veggies with the parmesan. Enjoy.

Cheesy Cauliflower

This makes four servings, and each serving contains 183 calories, 4 g net carbs, 15 g fat, and 8 g protein.

What you need:

- Pepper

- Salt

- Room temp butter, 2 tbsp.

- Heavy cream, .25 c

- Shredded cheddar, .5 c

- Roughly chopped cauliflower, 1 head

What you do:

1. Add water to a pot and fill three-quarters full. Place on high and bring to boil.

2. Add the cauliflower and blanch until tender, around five minutes. Drain the cauliflower.

3. Place the cauliflower in a food processor and add in the butter, cream, and cheese. Puree the mixture until it is whipped and creamy.

4. Season to taste with pepper and salt.

Cheesy Bacon Deviled Eggs

This makes 12 servings, and each serving contains 85 calories, 2 g net carbs, 7 g fat, and 6 g protein.

What you need:

- Chopped and cooked bacon, 6 slices

- Pepper

- Salt

- Dijon mustard, .5 tsp.

- Shredded Swiss cheese, .25 tsp.

- Chopped avocado, .25

- Mayonnaise, .25 c

- Hardboiled eggs, 6

What you do:

1. Cut the eggs in half lengthwise.

2. Remove the yolks carefully and put them in a bowl. Set the whites onto a plate.

3. Using a fork and mash the yolks. Add in the mustard, cheese, avocado, and mayonnaise. Stir well until blended. Season with pepper and salt.

4. Carefully spoon the yolk mixture into each egg white. Add chopped bacon onto the top of each egg.

5. If not eating immediately, store them in an airtight container in the refrigerator for no longer than one day.

Chapter 13: Desserts, Fat Bombs, and Extras

Doughnut Holes

This makes eight servings, and each serving contains 142 calories, 6.2 g net carbs, 14.1 g fat, and 0 g protein.

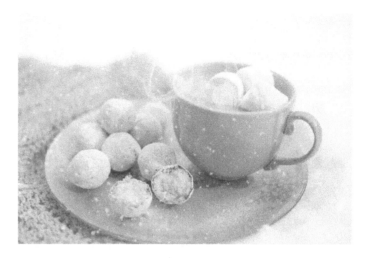

What you need:

- Vanilla extract, 1 tsp.

- Coconut flour, 1 tbsp.

- Coconut oil, 2 tbsp.

- Stevie, 2 tbsp.

- Hot water, 2 oz.

- Softened coconut butter, 4 oz.

What you do:

1. Set aside one tablespoon of sweetener. Place all of the rest of the ingredients into a mixer and combine until mixed thoroughly.

2. Place into the freezer for 30 minutes to allow it to set up.

3. Once it has hardened, divide it into eight portions and roll them into balls.

4. Add the reserved sweetener into a food processor and blend until it turns into powder.

5. Roll the balls into the powder and enjoy.

Chocolate-Coconut Treats

This makes 16 servings, and each serving contains 43 calories, 1 g net carbs, 5 g fat, and 1 g protein.

What you need:

- Shredded unsweetened coconut, .25 c

- Salt

- Liquid stevia, 4 drops

- Unsweetened cocoa powder, .25 c

- Coconut oil, .33 c

What you do:

1. Place some parchment paper in a 6-inch square baking dish and set aside.

2. In a pot, add in the salt, stevia, cocoa, and coconut oil. Stir everything together for about three minutes.

3. Mix in the coconut and press the mixture into the prepared baking dish.

4. Place in the fridge until it has hardened, around 30 minutes.

5. Cut into 16 equal squares and keep stored in a cool place.

Herbed Avocado Butter

This makes two cups, and one tablespoon contains 22 calories, 1 g net carbs, 2 g fat, and 0 g protein.

What you need:

- Pepper
- Salt
- Minced garlic, 1 tsp.
- Chopped basil, 1 tsp.
- Chopped cilantro, 2 tsp.
- Lemon juice, .5 of a lemon
- Quartered avocado, 1
- Room temp butter, .25 c

What you do:

1. Add the garlic, basil, cilantro, lemon juice, avocado, and butter to a food processor and mix up until it is smooth.
2. Season with some pepper and salt.
3. Place the butter on a sheet of wax paper and roll the compound butter into a log share. Place this back in the fridge until it is firm, around four hours.
4. You can use this on chicken, fish, or steak. Keep stored, wrapped tightly, in the freezer for a week.

Mayonnaise

This makes four cups, and two tablespoons contain 61 calories, 0 g net carbs, 7 g fat, and 0 g protein.

What you need:

- Pepper

- Salt

- Lemon juice, .25 c

- EVOO, 1.5 c

- Dijon mustard, 2 tbsp.

- Eggs, 2

What you do:

1. By Hand – place the mustard and eggs in a large bowl and whisk together until they are well combined, around two minutes.

2. Pour the oil into the eggs in a continuous thin stream as you continue to whisk. Do this until the mayonnaise is thick and emulsified.

3. Add in the lemon juice and whisk together until blended. Season with some pepper and salt.

4. With a Food Processor – add the mustard and eggs into a food processor and blend until smooth.

5. With the processor running, slowly drizzle in the oil, mixing until the mayonnaise is thick and emulsified.

6. Add in the lemon juice until smooth and season with some salt and pepper.

Peanut Butter Cups

This makes six servings, and each serving contains: 231 calories, 3 g net carbs, 15.1 g fat, and 2 g protein.

What you need:

- Vanilla, .25 tsp.

- Stevia, .5 tsp.

- Cocoa powder, 1 tbsp.

- Unsweetened baker's chocolate, 1 oz.

- Coconut oil, .25 c

- Peanut butter, .25 c

What you do:

1. In a pot, add the baker's chocolate and allow it to melt.

2. Mix in the peanut butter. The softer it is, the easier it will be to mix in. Stir in the cocoa powder and coconut oil until it is thoroughly mixed.

3. Using paper or silicone cupcake liners, pour the mixture into six cupcake molds.

4. Allow them to freeze for an hour to let it solidify. Once hard, you can take them out of the liners and store them, or leave them in the liners until you want to eat them. Keep them stored in the fridge.

Peanut Butter Mousse

This makes four servings, and each serving contains 280 calories, 3 g net carbs, 28 g fat, and 6 g protein.

What you need:

- Liquid stevia, 4 drops

- Vanilla, 1 tsp.

- Peanut butter, .25 c

- Heavy cream, 1 c

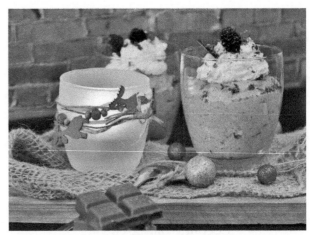

What you do:

1. Using a medium bowl, beat the peanut butter, heavy cream, stevia, and vanilla together until they form stiff peaks. This takes about five minutes.

2. Spoon the mousse into four bowls and refrigerate for at last 30 minutes before you serve.

Strawberry Butter

This makes three cups, and each tablespoon contains 23 calories, 1 g net carbs, 2 g fat, and 0 g protein.

What you need:

- Vanilla, 1 tsp.

- Fresh lemon juice, .5 tbsp.

- Fresh strawberries, .75 c

- Coconut oil, 1 tbsp.

- Shredded unsweetened coconut, 2 c

What you do:

1. Place the coconut in a food processor and puree it until it becomes smooth and buttery. This will take about 15 minutes.

2. Add in the vanilla, lemon juice, strawberries, and coconut oil to the coconut mixture. Process this until smooth. You will want to scrape the sides of the bowl down.

3. Pour the butter through a fine sieve to get rid of the strawberry seeds. You can use the back of a spoon to help push the butter through.

4. Place the strawberry butter in an airtight container and keep it refrigerated. It will last for at least two weeks.

5. This is great served on fish or chicken.

Balsamic Dressing

This makes one cup, and each tablespoon contains 83 calories, 0 g net carbs, 9 g fat, and 0 g protein.

What you need:

- Pepper

- Salt

- Minced garlic, 1 tsp.

- Chopped basil, 1 tsp.

- Chopped oregano, 2 tbsp.

- Balsamic vinegar, .25 c

- EVOO, 1 c

What you do:

1. Add the vinegar and olive oil to a bowl and whisk it together until they are well emulsified. This takes about three minutes.

2. Whisk in the garlic, basil, and oregano until it is well combined, around one minute.

3. Add in the pepper and salt to your taste.

4. Pour into an airtight container. This can be stored in the refrigerator for up to a week. Before you use it, shake it well.

Hollandaise

This makes two cups, and each tablespoon contains 173 calories, 1 g net carbs, 17 g fat, and 5 g protein.

What you need:

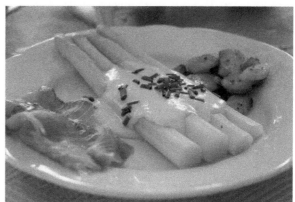

- Salt

- Lemon juice, 4 tsp.

- Cold water, 2 tsp.

- Egg yolks, 4

- Unsalted butter, 1.5 c

What you do:

1. Melt the butter in a heavy-bottomed pot on low heat.

2. Take the pot off the heat and allow the butter to cool for five minutes.

3. Carefully skim the foam from the top of the cooled butter.

4. Slowly add the clarified butter into a container, leave all of the milky solids in the bottom of the pot.

5. Discard these solids and allow the clarified butter to cool until just warm. This takes about 15 minutes.

6. Place a pot with about three inches of water on medium heat, heating until it simmers.

7. Using a stainless steel bowl, add in the yolks along with two teaspoons of cold water and whisk them together until they are foamy and light. This takes about three minutes.

8. Add in three or four drops of lemon juice to the yolk mixture and whisk it together for about a minute.

9. Set the bowl on top of the pot, making sure that the bottom of the bowl doesn't hit the water.

10. Whisk the mixture together until they thicken up, around one to two minutes. Set the bowl off of the simmering water.

11. In a very thin stream, add the clarified butter to the yolk mixture. You need to whisk continuously until you use all of the butter and the sauce is thick and smooth. If the butter is added too quickly, the sauce could end up breaking.

12. Whisk in the rest of the lemon juice and salt.

13. This sauce will have to be used right away or only let sit for an hour. Get rid of any that you don't use.

Conclusion

Thank you for making it through to the end of *Keto Diet for Beginners 2021*. Let's hope it was informative and able to provide you with all of the tools you need to achieve your goals, whatever they may be.

You now have all the information you need to begin a successful ketogenic diet. This is a wonderful diet to follow to lose weight and even to maintain your desired weight. While, at first, you may experience some negative side effects, they will go away if you stick with it. It may seem tough, but it's worth it. You will notice results nearly immediately. Now, it's time to get started.

Finally, if you found this book useful in any way, a review is always appreciated!

Description

Something that nearly every person can relate to is struggling to lose weight. This is true if you are looking to lose that stubborn five pounds or if you have a lot of weight to lose. It's frustrating, and there is a nauseating amount of weight loss plans out there. How is a person supposed to be able to figure out how to lose weight when the professionals aren't even sure?

That's where this book and the ketogenic diet come into play. With this book, you will learn everything that you need to know to start a ketogenic diet and lose weight for good. If you scour the internet, you will find a lot of different, conflicting information on the keto diet. Some say it's terrible, some are lukewarm about it, and others believe it is the best weight loss plan ever. Whatever side you take is up to you, but I'm hoping that, with this book, you will learn to love this diet.

In this book, you will learn:

- How to start a ketogenic diet

- A meal plan to help you lose 21 pounds in 21 days

- What ketosis is and why it's so important

- Lots of recipes so that you never go hungry

- The different ketogenic plans

- The side effects that can happen

- What you can eat

- And much more!

The ketogenic diet is more than a weight loss plan. It's a way of life that brings so many more benefits than other weight loss plans. While you may find it difficult when you start the diet, it does get easier. The payoff is worth the effort. Don't wait any longer and get started today.